DATE DUE

JUL 2 1 1994	
APR 1 1 1995	
DEC 1 4 1995	
FEB - 3 1996	
AUG 1 6 2001	

BRODART   Cat. No. 23-221

Drum and Stethoscope

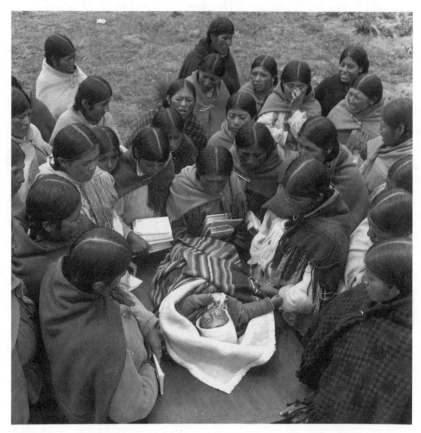

Midwife teaching Aymara women childcare in Peñas, Bolivia.

Drum and Stethoscope

Integrating Ethnomedicine and Biomedicine
in Bolivia

JOSEPH W. BASTIEN

University of Utah Press
Salt Lake City

∞ This symbol indicates books printed on paper that meets the mini-
mum requirements of American National Standard for Information
Services—Permanence of Paper for Printed Library Materials, ANSI
A39.38-1984.

Cover illustration by Bailey-Montague & Associates, Salt Lake City

LIBRARY OF CONGRESS CATALOGING-IN-PUBLICATION DATA

Bastien, Joseph William, 1935–
    Drum and stethoscope : integrating ethnomedicine and
biomedicine in Bolivia / Joseph W. Bastien.
        p.   cm.
    Includes bibliographical references and index.
    ISBN 0-87480-386-1
    1. Medical care—Bolivia. 2. Folk medicine—Bolivia. I. Title.
    [DNLM: 1. Delivery of Health Care—Bolivia. 2. Medicine,
Herbal—Bolivia. 3. Medicine, Traditional—Bolivia.
WA 395 B326d]
RA461.B37 1992
362.1'042'0984—dc20
DNLM/DLC   92-53602
for Library of Congress   CIP

For my mother
MARY MAGDELEN ARENDT BASTIEN
(1892–1972)
who cured me of polio when I was three years old
after being told by doctors that I would never walk again
to which she replied
"Only God determines that!"

Contents

Preface

This book provides ethnographic examples of ways in which ethno-medical healers can collaborate with doctors and nurses to improve the health of peasants in regions of the undeveloped world. Many of the examples are from the Aymara and Quechua speakers of the Andes where I have conducted fieldwork from 1963 to the present. The following is a case in point.

In August 1989 I had returned from the mountains, where I was doing fieldwork, because of a swollen and very sore throat. In the rarefied atmosphere of 13,000 feet I had difficulty breathing. I went to an integrated clinic that offers biomedicine and ethnomedicine, located on Calle Santa Cruz of La Paz, Bolivia. As I walked through the doorway, a woman doctor greeted me. She introduced herself as Alicia and then carefully examined me, taking my blood pressure, counting my pulse, and questioning me about my sore throat. She concluded that I had strep throat and gave me some penicillin. Figuring this would cure me, I began to leave when she recommended that I talk with the Kallawaya herbalist in the adjacent office. Alicia introduced me to this herbalist, Lucas Ortiz, who asked a different set of questions: What had I been doing? At what altitudes had I been living? What had I been drinking? And what was I eating? Lucas felt my pulse more thoroughly than Alicia. Collecting a urine sample, he held it in front of the window to reflect the rays of the sun and looked for telltale images. He then prescribed *luriwichu* (*Mutisia acuminata* R. & P.) to be taken as a tea three times a day. He also told me to gargle with salt water every hour and to drink a glass of warm lemon juice with a shot of pisco before going to bed. And to be on the safe side, Lucas had me see Jaime Zalles, a doctor trained in homeopathic and naturalistic medicine. Jaime recommended that I use the steam-bath treatment in an adjacent room. He also said that I should return on another occasion to complete the homeopathic treatment.

After I had recovered, I talked with patients of this clinic. They ranged from wealthy Bolivians to poor peasants. Several provided testimonies of why they liked this clinic and how they had been cured. One Indian woman spent upwards of an hour describing how desperate she had been before coming to this clinic. Bolivians frequented this clinic because it combined ethnomedicine with bio-medicine, taking as it were the best from a long tradition of Andean medicine with herbalists and other specialists and combining this with the biomedicine of doctors and nurses. This clinic is one ex-ample of what is being done in Bolivia and other parts of the world to integrate practitioners of biomedicine and ethnomedicine.

Most of the information in this book is taken from my experience in working as a medical anthropologist among doctors and nurses in Bolivia. As an advisor to health projects I have also found ways to use available resources to improve the health of Bolivians. The most available resource was the rich Andean medical tradition of herbal-ists, shamans, ritualists, bonesetters, diviners, masseurs, and other indigenous specialists. The biggest obstacle to ethnomedicine was the resistance of doctors and nurses toward these practitioners. There was, and still is, in Bolivia and other parts of the world the belief, especially on the part of government officials, that doctors and pharmacists should do away with *curanderos*, shamans, midwives, and herbalists with regard to health projects.

Since 1981 I have given workshops to doctors, nurses, midwives, herbalists, shamans, and diviners to foment cooperation and inte-gration between practitioners of biomedical and ethnomedical tra-ditions. The goal of the workshops was to get the doctors to accept regional medical traditions as part of an integrated health plan for Bolivia.

As for terms, the "biomedical tradition" refers to that practiced by doctors and is based on the pathogenic causes for illnesses as supported by microbiology (Pillsbury 1979). Biomedicine is some-times called "Western" and "modern" medicine, which is misleading because it extends beyond the Western world and is traditional (Crandon-Malamud 1987:473). Doctors assume that biomedicine is the most advanced and correct way to heal because of its reputed scientific basis and that it is universal and more accurately attuned to human physiology than are alternative medical systems.

The "ethnomedical system" refers to healing practices that have arisen as a folk tradition peculiar to the people of a given region, and for this reason it is also called "regional" medicine. Ethnomedi-cine derives from ways in which native practitioners adapt to ill-nesses using available resources. Ethnomedicine is also an ethnosci-ence that includes modern and traditional practices as well as empirical investigation and conceptual theories. Native healers con-tend that their practices cure because of experience, a knowledge of plants, and the ability to understand and to regulate the relationship of the ailing person with the environment and the universe.

As a result of the workshops in Oruro, practitioners of biomedical and ethnomedical traditions began to talk and cooperate in Bolivia with some interesting results. This has been fortunate for biomedicine, because Bolivia as well as many other countries throughout the world—such as China with its combination of barefoot doctors, herbalists, and acupuncturists—is incorporating biomedicine and its technology within the regional medical traditions. In Bolivia and elsewhere this movement toward an articulated model of health care recognizes deep cultural patterns of continuity in ethnomedicine. It also increases available medical care.

Metaphorically, one can understand an integration of biomedical and ethnomedical traditions as analogous to a flood and a river. Biomedicine is the flood inundating cities and rural areas with antibiotics, vaccinations, insecticides, clinics, hospitals, and doctors and nurses (not to imply, however, its availability to peasants, but rather its influential presence). Ethnomedicine is like the underground streams, the dried-out arroyos, and the rivers with deep channels that merge and form into vast waterways, the floods of different times and regions. When it occurs, the flood washes away the old riverbed until slowly the water once again begins to flow according to the channels of the river (see Gavin Smith 1989:17).

The integration of ethnomedicine and biomedicine does not imply that modern medicine should return to past medicinal practices, but rather that it should include the many beneficial and adaptive practices that ethnomedicine has to offer. Thus the sick can utilize resources and diagnoses from the roots and branches of ethnomedical and biomedical traditions. Cultures are not isolated entities, like fishbowls, separated from each other, but are rather concentric circles of overlapping spheres of influence. Especially now, travelers, television, and telephones invade the corners of the world, and "natives" frequent the metropolises (Clifford 1988). This conjuncture also takes place in biomedical and ethnomedical traditions as the past and present, the cosmopolitan and regional, come together with doctors and healers uniting to cure universal suffering.

Another reason for this study is that ethnomedical systems provide viable alternatives to costly biomedical systems, especially now when the resources of the universe are rapidly being depleted. At the Second International Conference of Ethnobiology in Kunming,

China, in 1990, the delegates unanimously agreed that for the preservation of ethnic populations and native plants and animals, it is necessary to study and preserve ethnosciences from all regions of the world. What were once thought to be outdated and irrelevant folklores are now being "salvaged" to recover ways of healing a patient of the universe, our world. The purpose of this book is to present ethnographic descriptions of instances in Bolivia where biomedicine has integrated with ethnomedicine as well as to evaluate areas where it has not and to suggest possible avenues of collaboration. Its relevance is to present ways in which collaboration between biomedicine and ethnomedicine can be accomplished in other parts of the world. Because ethnomedical practitioners constitute the major health resource for peoples of rural and undeveloped areas, their collaboration with doctors and nurses is necessary to improve world health.

Drawing on ethnographic data on the orientation and training of physicians and nurses to accept ethnomedical practices and to communicate with ethnomedical healers in Bolivia (and drawing further on data from other parts of the world pertaining to this issue), this book offers suggestions on what should be the criteria for selection of practitioners, who should set them, what folk specialists should be integrated into the national health-care system, and what training is necessary to accomplish this.

Part I deals with practical and theoretical issues involved in integrating biomedicine and ethnomedicine: the high incidence of illnesses in undeveloped countries, where ethnomedical practitioners are the basic health resource; the persistence of ethnic concepts of disease and ethnomedical practices; the limited success of primary health-care programs throughout the world; and the objections by doctors to the practices of indigenous healers. Chapter 1 describes the deficiencies of biomedicine in providing primary health care for peasants of the developing world. Without ethnomedical practitioners and community participation, primary health care will not meet the objectives set forth by the World Health Organization. Chapter 2 analyzes the advantages and disadvantages of ethnomedicine. An articulated model of integration between biomedical and ethnomedical practitioners, which takes into account some objections that doctors have to ethnomedicine, is presented.

Part II contains ethnographic accounts of the adaptive strategies that ethnomedical practitioners have devised and the conflicts they have with biomedical practitioners. Chapter 3 includes an analysis of the ethnomedical system of Kallawaya herbalists in Bolivia and how they have adapted to biomedicine in the twentieth century. Emphasis is placed on three contemporaneous herbalists and their strategies to articulate with biomedicine. Chapter 4 is about psychosocial healing, specifically shamanism. Various explanations of its reputed efficacy in healing are discussed, and a case study is presented on the conflict between a shaman and an auxiliary nurse in Qaqachaka, Bolivia. The case study describes how a shaman tries to incorporate a practitioner of biomedicine into his ethnomedical system. The shaman's ritual demonstrates the place of catharsis and group therapy in healing. It also illustrates the political factors involved with the joint therapy of biomedical and ethnomedical practitioners.

Part III covers the strategy of ethnomedical practitioners as mediators between ethnomedicine and biomedicine. Chapter 5 is about community health workers and how they serve as mediators between biomedicine and ethnomedicine. It describes how government and private-agency-sponsored outreach programs with community health workers in Guatemala and Bolivia utilize members of the dominant medical establishments to elicit community participation in integrated primary health-care programs. Chapter 6 deals with midwives and their integration with biomedicine. Most numerous of ethnomedical practitioners, midwives deliver the majority of babies in rural communities of Asia, Africa, and Latin America, areas with high perinatal infant mortality. Problems discussed in this chapter focus on educating doctors to collaborate with midwives and on training courses for midwives in Bolivia. This chapter also contains cross-cultural comparisons of the biomedical integration of midwives in other parts of the world.

Part IV concerns training biomedical practitioners in the understanding of ethnomedicine and in how to collaborate with ethnomedical practitioners in a coordinated strategy. Chapter 7 is about how doctors and nurses collaborate with ethnomedical practitioners in joint therapy for culturally defined illnesses. Training courses for biomedical and ethnomedical practitioners assist them in understanding each other's systems. Integrated clinics with biomedical and ethnomedical practitioners facilitate joint therapy, especially for patients desiring holistic healing. Chapter 8 examines cross-cultural concepts of neonatal tetanus and how this knowledge can be used for vaccinations with tetanus toxoid. The pervasive problem of biomedicine is how to communicate to peasants its complex technology within their cultural terms. As a result, doctors and nurses frequently omit explanations about vaccinations and diseases and just line people up to receive the "silver bullet." Ethnomedical practitioners can assist in immunization campaigns by helping doctors and nurses understand the different concepts and then translating them into medically relevant terms for members of the community.

The concluding chapter contains a summary of practical applications of how to articulate biomedicine and ethnomedicine on the national level. In addition to recognition, respect, and rewards, essential to the articulation of ethnomedicine with biomedicine is a functioning system of health records and referrals.

The value in reading this book is to learn more about the role of ethnomedicine in world health, to understand the concrete ways integration has been achieved in Bolivia, and to have access to improved methods for health programs in other countries. In addition to its applied value, this book also reveals the role of ethnomedicine in the healing process. It introduces a coordinated strategy to incorporate biomedicine and ethnomedicine.

There is much talk in development circles these days about "grass-roots" or "bottom-up" development. If this talk proves to be serious, then this work suggests how this might be done in the health sector.

Acknowledgments

Numerous friends and colleagues have helped me with various aspects of this work, and it is with pleasure that I acknowledge their assistance. I am especially grateful to the following: The graduate dean at the University of Texas, Bob Perkins, provided me with research stipends. The president of Wenner-Gren Foundation for Anthropological Research, Sydel Silverman, awarded me funds to do research in 1987 and 1988. Grants curator Ann Berg also assisted me.

Cassandra A. Pyle, executive director of the Council for International Exchange of Scholars, and Dr. Charles W. Dunn, chairman for the J. William Fulbright foreign scholarships, awarded me a grant for the 1991–92 Fulbright program in anthropology and archaeology, making continued fieldwork in Bolivia possible. Rosemary Lyon, CIES program officer; Cynthia Wolloch, United States Information Agency program officer; and Robert Callahan and Kimberly King, officers of the United States Information Services, helped me while I was in Bolivia.

While Bolivian ambassador from 1988 to 1991, Robert Gelbard contributed greatly to an understading of Aymara and Quechua cultures by promoting archaeological investigations in Tiahuanaco and supporting ethnomedical studies. His efforts facilitated my research in Bolivia. Under his leadership and that of Paul Hartenberger, chief of the Health and Humanitarian Division of the United States Agency for International Development/Bolivia, articulation of bio- and ethnomedicine has improved in Bolivia.

The National Institute of Health awarded me and my coinvestigators, Manfred Reinecke of Texas Christian University and W. Edward Robinson of the University of California at Irvine, a grant, "Testing of Anti-HIV Compounds from Medicinal Plants," for the years 1991 until 1994. This grant supports the study of Kallawaya ethnopharmacology as well as the active ingredients in the plants.

In Bolivia, Wally Chastain provided me with a vehicle, friendship, and valuable information. Robert Steinglass assisted me in the design of the neonatal tetanus research in Bolivia. Paul Hartenberger, Rafael Indaburu, and Joel Kuritsky instructed me about public health measures and primary health care in Bolivia. Michelle

Fryer, Tom Tilson, Filemon Heredia, and Alvaro Cisneros assisted me in deriving conclusions about cross-cultural education.

The Kallawaya of Province Bautista Saavedra allowed me to live with them for a year in 1972 and numerous summers thereafter. I am most indebted to herbalists Florentino Alvarez, Nestor Llaves, and Mario Salcedo for providing me with knowledge about their ethnomedicine.

Community health workers in the Department of Oruro, Bolivia, allowed me to work with them during summers from 1982 until 1985. Their participation in training courses on ethnomedicine and biomedicine that Dr. Oscar Velasco, Angela Lutena, and I directed provided me with practical ways of integrating biomedicine and ethnomedicine.

Gregory Rake invited me in 1981 to work with him in starting a community-health-worker program and in establishing an integrated primary health-care system for the Ministry of Health in the Department of Oruro. Rake's relentless efforts were a constant motivation to me in our shared conviction that biomedical and ethnomedical practioners need to work together. The director of education for the same project, Angela Lutena, exhibited remarkable cross-cultural skills in health education.

Among my colleagues in medical anthropology, Oscar Velasco demonstrated in his medical practice as a doctor how to incorporate ethnomedicine with biomedicine. As director of traditional medicine in Oruro and working jointly with herbalists, midwives, and shamans in an integrated clinic, Velasco showed other Bolivian doctors how to articulate ethnomedicine with biomedicine. Oscar Velasco and Javier Palazuelos assisted in the neonatal tetanus study in Bolivia. Relentless research assistants, Velasco and Palazuelos aided greatly in collection of data and analysis. Graduate students in medical anthropology at the University of Texas in Arlington, Henry Migala coauthored chapter 2, and Nancy Edens coauthored chapter 6. Professor of anthropology at the University of Victoria, Ross Crumrine suggested revisions for this book. Lynn Bauman proofed and edited the manuscript. Timothy Wright critically reviewed the manuscript and provided many corrections. I especially thank Libbet Crandon-Malamud, whose critical review, scholarly contributions, and encouragement helped me finish this book.

Secretaries Kathy Rowe, Jane Nicol, Ange Moyer, and Margaret Beseda typed and proofed the manuscript. Felix Espinoza drove me safely over 8,000 miles of unpaved roads in Bolivia without getting lost, always arriving on schedule. My home away from home in La

Paz, Bolivia, is the house of Maria and Pedro Cabanillos, who receive me like a brother. Also, my friends Michele and Mat Cheney frequently gave of their hospitality and food. These friendships and kindnesses have provided me with the emotional support necessary throughout thirty years of fieldwork in the Andes.

Most of all, the Bolivian people always greet me as a friend. They share themselves with me and love me. The most felicitous event of my life was my going to Bolivia in Juen 1963. Although I have returned to the States many times, I always want to go back to Bolivia. *Viva Bolivia!*

As an anthropologist with a family, I cherish greatly the support of my wife, Judy, who always encourages me to do research even though it means long absences and assuming my duties in the family. My children, Suzanne, Brian, and Kristin, missed me at times when they needed me, yet they also supported me. Absence from loved ones is the most difficult part of fieldwork, and it is unbearable without their understanding and support. My love for you, wherever you are, is my thank you.

To the above, and others forgotten, a toast of gratitude: may your contributions to this book not go unnoticed, and in the event that people suffer less and are healed, may you be given credit.

PART I
Articulation of Biomedicine and Ethnomedicine

OBJECTIVES, PROBLEMS, AND STRATEGIES

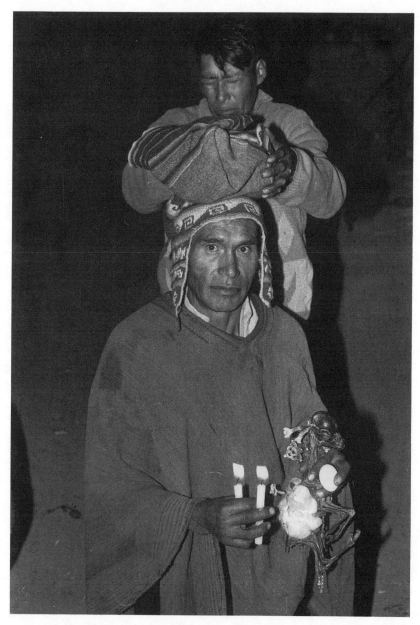

Curandero placing bundle of ritual food on Marcelino Yanahuaya's head in ritual to cure two-year-old Erminia Yanahuaya. Food was to feed the earth shrines
of *ayllu* Kaata. The llama fetus is a central symbol for the earth shrines.

1

Biomedical Centrism

DEFICIENCIES OF BIOMEDICINE IN PRIMARY HEALTH CARE*

Many physicians, policy makers, and scholars contend that biomedicine is the only solution to the primary health-care needs of developing countries. They fail to recognize that ethnomedical practitioners are important health resources for the developing world, where biomedical practitioners have encountered a number of problems in providing primary health care.

Throughout the developing world, sickness and malnutrition persistently plague the rapidly growing population. Relying exclusively on biomedicine, international and national health agencies have not been able to meet adequately these people's health needs. Making matters worse by disregarding ethnomedicine, health planners consider a community without doctors and nurses devoid of health care. This attitude is one of biomedical centrism because its proponents refuse to see that each culture has its own complex and adaptive methodologies for coping with illnesses. These theoretical systems explain the occurrence of illness and disease based on the secular and religious beliefs of the culture, and it is in these systems that the people place their confidence first and foremost.

Ethnomedicine, with its native healers, such as herbalists, healers, ritualists, and midwives, constitutes basic health systems for many villages and cities throughout the world. Its practitioners form the core of primary health-care workers in up to 90 percent of rural populations in developing countries. Midwives still deliver about 90 percent of all infants in these countries (Pillsbury 1979:vii–viii). In urban communities, biomedical practice has moved in alongside the traditional health system, and ethnomedical practitioners find they have new and more frequent opportunities to operate successfully in a biomedical environment. Success in either medical system is often dependent on the attitudes and responses of patients; belief in and acceptance of either practice is important in the curing process. The persistence of ethnic concepts of disease and medical practices

* Henri Migala assisted with research for this chapter.

3

in an urban setting indicates that ethnomedicine offers something the local population finds important (see Alvarado 1978). It is primarily for this subjective reasoning, and also due to certain objective realities, that any health program planned for a developing area (or an urban setting where there is a population that still adheres to regional medical ideologies) requires at least the collaboration, and ideally the integration, of both biomedical and ethnomedical beliefs and practices. However practical this proposal may be, certain objections have been raised concerning the recognition and utilization of ethnomedical practitioners and practices.

Although biomedicine has significant contributions to make, it is at a disadvantage when confronted with patients who do not associate it with their belief system. Medical efficacy alone is not sufficient to ensure its adoption nor is it necessarily the most significant aspect of any medical system (Crandon-Malamud 1991).

Primary Health Care

Ethnomedical practitioners were officially recognized as important for international health when the World Health Organization (WHO) at the Alma-Ata conference in 1978 and the Pan American Health Organization (PAHO) throughout the 1970s and 1980s emphasized primary health care (PHC) as a priority in developing countries. The director-general of WHO and the executive director of UNICEF issued a joint report at the International Conference on Primary Health Care, Alma-Ata, USSR, with the following text:

> 82. Traditional medical practitioners and birth attendants are found in most societies. They are part of the local community, culture and traditions, and continue to have high social standing in many places, exerting considerable influence on local health practices. With the support of the formal health system, these indigenous practitioners can become important allies in organizing efforts to improve the health of the community. Some communities may select them as community health workers. It is therefore well worthwhile exploring the possibilities of engaging them in primary health care and of training them accordingly. (WHO and UNICEF 1978:33)

Primary health care is defined as essential health care made universally accessible to individuals and families in the community by means available to them, through their full participation and at a cost that the community and country can afford (WHO and UNICEF 1978:2–3). And ethnomedical practitioners and community health workers (CHWs) are necessary in this effort. The goals of the primary health-care program are to bring basic health care to underserved rural regions of the country, with emphasis on reducing infant mortality and infectious disease rates; improving nutrition, hygiene, and sanitation; "first-aid" treatment of maladies; and increasing life expectancy (see Coreil and Mull 1990; Phillips 1190:150–77).

As the Alma-Ata report states, to make primary health care universally accessible in the community as quickly as possible, maximum community and individual self-reliance for health development would be essential. In order to attain such self-reliance, full community participation would be necessary in the planning, organization, and management of any primary health-care system (WHO and UNICEF 1978:2; see also Morgan 1989:233). Thus, planners wanted to avoid implementation of primary health care as a unilateral imposition of biomedicine by outsiders upon the health problems of the community.

This emphasis on the utilization of ethnomedicine and community participation in primary health care created problems for international health agencies. Following these guidelines, health planners not only had to integrate ethnomedicine with biomedicine but also had to consider the political wills of individuals, their communities, and countries.

Fourteen years after the WHO resolution concerning ethnomedical practitioners, community health workers, and community participation, primary health-care systems in many countries still do not include ethnomedical practitioners—not even midwives (Green 1988; MacCormack 1986). Doctors and nurses infrequently support ethnomedical programs; few national drug policies have been revised to support ethnomedicines; and governments seldom sponsor ethnomedical programs and rarely provide training courses for ethnomedical practitioners (Velimirovic 1990:51–78). Relative success has been achieved through the training of community health workers, but this, too, has been met with fierce political resistance. CHW programs were successful because of low attrition, high community utilization, lowered mortality, and low costs.

Within the social sciences, the integrated primary health-care approach has its supporters (e.g., Bryant 1980; Donahue 1990; Jordan 1990; Mull 1990; Welsch 1988), its thoughtful critics (e.g., de Kadt 1982; Gish 1979; Velimirovic 1990), and its detractors (e.g., Navarro 1984; Ugalde 1985), all identifying in their own way some of its problems and possibilities. They all agree, however, that the Alma-Ata declaration is an extremely difficult (if not impossible) policy to put into practice (Welsch 1988:1): ideology and reality conflict in the vacuum of ideas to operationalize it.

Boris Velimirovic (1990:72) criticizes anthropologists for enthusiastically endorsing the Alma-Ata document because it seems to promote the maintenance of cultural diversity in ethnomedicine for its own sake. To support ethnomedicine for its own sake is not an objective of this book; ethnomedicine should be viewed as a logical alternative and adaptive strategy that is readily available and accessible for peoples throughout the developing world. The use of ethnomedicine should not be seen as a substitute for biomedicine in solving the problems of insufficient health-care coverage. Ethnomedicine, like biomedicine, has several possibilities: its practitioners sometimes cure because of physical causality, at other times they promote the healing process through indirect effects (psychosocial, environmental, and cultural), and at still other times they have no effect and even damage the person's health. Medical anthropologists are not interested in romanticizing ethnomedicine, but rather in investigating its beneficial possibilities, in assisting ethnomedical practitioners to eradicate harmful practices, and in illustrating to doctors and nurses how the positive aspects of ethnomedicine can fit into primary health care. As Michael Tan (1988:10) concludes, the principles of primary health care as expressed by the World Health Organization are still crucial: recognition and development of local resources through actual immersion in the community and the encouragement of people's participation.

Deficiencies in the Biomedical Model of Healing and Primary Health Care

During the 1950s and 1960s international health workers believed that biomedicine would revolutionize world health with its universally applicable scientific methods, but as the World Health Organization later recognized, this never came to pass. Based on molecular biology, biomedicine posits that diseases are explained as deviations from the norms of measurable biological variables (Engel 1977:129–36). Social, cultural, and behavioral factors are not considered significant causes of disease in this mechanistic, physiological model. Unusual behavior connected with illness is explained as the product of disordered processes. Consequently, biomedical practitioners treat disease as an independent biological entity (Medalie 1978; in Kleinman 1978:94).

In contrast, the Kallawaya ethnomedical model does not make a

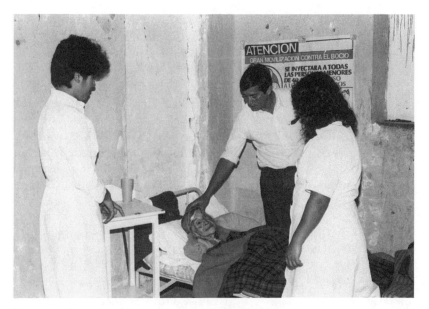

Doctor and nurses taking care of a patient in Bolivia.

distinction between measurable deviance from expected biological functioning and not feeling well (see Bastien 1987; Scrimshaw and Burleigh 1978). This model often defines illness, distinct from disease, in a social sense as interference with normal social behavior and the ability of the individual to work. Kallawaya medicine also differs from biomedicine in that the possible causes of disease may include problems or imbalances in the supernatural realm, body fluids, emotions, and the social or physical environment (Bastien 1987). Ethnomedicine interweaves illness, health maintenance, religion, and social relations (Scrimshaw and Burleigh 1978:30–31). These differences exist at essential levels of all ethnomedical ideologies and create problems in cross-cultural communication between practitioners of biomedical and ethnomedical systems.

Another obstacle to integration of the two approaches is that biomedical and ethnomedical systems are embedded in social classes. Higher-class physicians refer to their "biomedical culture" as a privileged system of discourse that attempts domination over ailing bodies and healers, whose ethnomedicine is an indicator of their lower social class. Since both ethnomedical and biomedical systems employ mechanisms of technology and meticulous rituals through which power is actually directed toward the body (see Foucault in Dreyfus and Rabinow 1983:113), it frequently happens that the sick person's body becomes an arena where the domination and resistance of social classes by doctors and native healers is played out (see Scheper-Hughes and Lock 1987; van Binsbergen 1988).

Doctors and nurses are often socially, culturally, and economically distant from rural people and consequently are aloof, condescending, disrespectful, and unsympathetic to the fact that in rural areas ill health is but one aspect of life where social classes, domination, and the intertwined problems of poverty exist (Pillsbury 1979:2). The existence of class distinction further exacerbates patient-healer relations when there is cultural distance—when the organization, practitioners, and procedures of biomedicine differ from customary beliefs about diseases and their causes, values, symbols, and behavior.

Modernization and development are drastically changing traditional ways of managing health in Bolivia and other developing countries. What has been lacking, however is an adequate way to deal with the social costs of biomedical technology and its effects on the social system into which it is introduced (Jordan 1990:114–15). Incorporation of biomedicine into cultural and social systems of developing countries necessitates the use of technologies socially acceptable and appropriate to their level of development. Ethnomedical practitioners can provide an appropriate, acceptable, and available resource for incorporating biomedicine into the community so that social and cultural values of the community are not disrupted.

Problems of social cost and "cultural and social distance" between practitioners of biomedicine and ethnomedicine are worldwide phenomena. In the United States, Kunitz (1983:130) observes that the Navajo healing system persists with remarkable internal consistency across a reservation the size of West Virginia and that the ceremonies and normative beliefs are practically identical with those documented at the turn of the century. There is little evidence that Navajos have incorporated new concepts or curing techniques into their ethnomedicine. One reason for this adherence to traditional beliefs is the Navajos' resistance to white dominance in general.

Before the 1950s the Navajos looked upon hospitals and sanatoria as houses of death, where it was almost certain the patient would contract ghost sickness. Today, however, as the rate of cure has improved, Navajos have come to accept the hospital, especially in the treatment of tuberculosis. Ceremonialists may even tell patients to do what the white doctors say instead of telling them to stay away at all costs (Kunitz 1983:131). The Navajos provide one example of an integrated health-care system that respects the differences and utilizes the resources of both biomedicine and ethnomedicine.

In Latin America, problems of "cultural and social distance" between biomedicine and ethnomedicine have been identified in Guatemala by Richard Adams (1952), Benjamin and Lois Paul (1975), and Carroll Behrhorst (1975, 1983) and in Mexico by Jack Brown (1963), Kaja Finkler (1985), James Young (1981), and Susan Scrimshaw and Elizabeth Burleigh (1978). A world leader in bringing health to peasants through biomedicine, Behrhorst (1983:xvii) writes of his first experiences in Guatemala as a doctor:

> We had to challenge some of the sacred institutions of modern medicine in order to meet the needs of the people on their own terms. Having reformulated the concept of "hospital," we now went on to challenge "the doctor" himself . . . [because] the vast majority of patients are in no real need of a sophisticated doctor—poor areas, such as rural Guatemala, plainly cannot afford the myth at all.

Behrhorst faced these problems by training responsible Indians from Guatemalan communities how to recognize and alleviate common medical problems. Up until civil war erupted in Guatemala, these health promoters were dealing with urgent health needs in fifty medically neglected communities. Tragically, the program is no longer operating.

The success of health promoters in Guatemala (in the past) and other parts of the world is that they are able to bridge the gap between biomedicine and ethnomedicine. Rural people, by a set of circumstances, depend on natural processes and nontechnical interventions to achieve health. Industrialized people view health within the context of physical procedures, technology, and chemically based remedies. "Whereas rural people," writes Behrhorst (1983: xxxiii), "stress their dependence on 'spirit' and on balanced relationships with fellow human beings and with nature, modern medicine largely discards these natural elements in favor of more elaborate techniques amenable to strict measurement and technical application." Health promoters serve as intermediaries between doctors and native healers; they understand and are sensitive to cultural traditions and the felt needs of the rural poor. The stronger the orientation of a health program toward these factors, the more successful the program is likely to be.

Doctors and nurses frequently do not know how to talk with peasants about diseases and health. In a study of biomedical health services among Hispanic communities along the border towns of the southern United States, Scrimshaw and Burleigh (1978:35) found that biomedically trained health-care providers are frustrated with non-compliance to prescribed treatment and a high morbidity rate among Mexican and Mexican American patients. They describe their patients as being concerned only with the present. Delay in treatment is seen as neglect or stupidity, and faith in God is considered fatalistic, passive, and apathetic. Doctors and nurses make little effort to understand ethnomedicine, which they characterize as being magic, irrational, and inferior to biomedicine. They become frustrated in the failure to communicate cross-culturally. Reciprocally, Mexican American patients view doctors with mistrust out of resistance to Anglo authority and power. They fear discrimination and criticism and suspect that the doctor is more interested in money than in their welfare. They consider biomedicine ineffective because doctors rely on technological "gadgets" for diagnosis, ignore supernatural factors, and subject them to lengthy treatments.

Frequently, biomedicine is incompatible with the beliefs, values, and behavior of rural people. Throughout the world, these people have culturally distinct ethnomedical systems that are based on assumptions about how the body works and how it is influenced by others, the environment, and the supernatural. These perceptions influence their values and behavior regarding medical treatment. For instance, nurses in Bolivia have difficulty convincing people to use oral rehydration therapy for diarrhea because of a belief that diarrhea is a wet disease which should be cured by using dry medicines (Bastien 1985). In another instance in Curva, Bolivia, herbalists refused to use an alcohol massage for a person with a high fever because they classified alcohol as a hot remedy. For these Bolivians, as well as for many other people in Latin America, health requires a balance of the hot, cold, wet, and dry in the body, with disease resulting from an imbalance of these qualities, which need to be equilibrated (Foster 1978, 1987). Less obvious are differences in values, such as treatment in the home with the family present rather than alone in the clinic, delivery of babies by midwives, and the refusal of women—out of modesty—to be examined by male doctors.

Doctors in developing countries have little success convincing people who are not educated in the ways of science about the causal relationships between illnesses and medically maladaptive behavior, especially when these individuals are routinized in another medical tradition and lack healthy alternatives. An obvious example is teaching children to wash with soap when they live where water and soap are scarce. Even in industrialized countries, doctors and nurses have a difficult time changing behavioral patterns of people regarding disease. People do not consider the effort of prevention to outweigh the benefits of indulgence even when they fully comprehend the consequences of these actions, such as smoking cigarettes, promiscuous sex, drinking alcohol, and fast driving.

In most parts of the developing world, the "cultural distance" between ethnomedicine and biomedicine is further compounded by a history of colonialism. The cultural circumstances of colonialism shaped the conceptual, professional, and political dimensions of Western medicine so that in the process of its transmission abroad, it acquired a new dimension, acting both as a cultural agent in itself and as an agent of Western expansion (MacLeod 1988:1). Many people of Kenya, for example, still consider biomedicine as foreign as the white faces, coats, and buildings associated with it. Such people are expected to have faith in something alien to them, a faith in something that has failed them in the past (Mburu 1977:158).

Under colonialism, the physician was a member of the bandwagon that played patriotic tunes favoring colonial rule. Colonial physicians in Africa and in other colonial empires labeled ethnomedicine as black magic, witch hunting, native superstition, primitive, or any other term that denigrated the local population and indirectly provided esteem and dominance to a colonial biomedicine that predominately treated whites and the native elite essential to their empire.

This critical view of colonial biomedicine cuts deeply into the study of medicine as being the heroic intervention against disease. A foremost world expert on vector disease control, Andy Arata (pers. com. 23 November 1990), says that the tropical diseases (malaria, yellow fever, dengue, encephalitis, leishmaniasis, and flukes) listed in 1890 continue to plague natives of the tropics endemically in the 1990s because peoples of these regions are poor and cannot afford to buy remedies. Consequently, insufficient research monies from pharmaceutical companies have gone into the eradication of these vector-borne diseases.

Biomedical therapeutics replacing ethnomedical therapeutics is not the reason for success in primary health care throughout the developing world. Rather, advances of the last century in nutrition, housing, and sanitation have had the greatest impact on rural populations. As practiced, biomedicine is a cultural institution, typically of Western culture, and is embedded in contemporary political and social thought (see Brock 1984; Stein 1990). As MacLeod (1988:1) forcefully writes:

As a cultural institution, biomedicine has the power to redefine (or "medicalize") concepts into the terms of its own discourse. Thus "medical imperialism", in the colloquialism of our day, now encompasses not only the conquest of new diseases but also the extension of what has been called the biomedical model over the ethnomedical world. It also implies the extension of Western cultural values to the non-West.

Nevertheless, although biomedical practices have reinforced dependence on colonial or neocolonial powers and sustained political hegemonies in the past, they do not create them. It is possible to disengage the science and art of biomedical healing from these colonial or neocolonial, inequitable, and hegemonic trappings so that the benefits of modern science can meet the challenges of hunger, poverty, ethnicity, racism, and disease. In part, this book, as well as the endeavors of other medical anthropologists, proposes ways that the scientific aspects of biomedicine can interrelate with the values and practices of ethnomedicine.

Economics of Health Care in Developing Countries

In addition to those described above, other practical limitations of the reliance on biomedicine for rural areas of the world are cost, personnel, change, and incompatibility. In general, biomedicine, even when limited to primary health care, is capital- rather than labor-intensive (Bastien 1982a). It is an expensive support system, with laboratories, clinics, and hospitals staffed by highly skilled personnel who have been trained in costly medical schools. The problem with a capital-intensive health delivery system is that it functions best in industrial countries or in cities where there is an accumulation of capital and a stable economy. Even though the facilities may have been donated by industrial countries, the operation of biomedical laboratories in major cities of developing countries drains these nations' health budgets and thus results in even poorer service to rural populations. As a product of industrial society, biomedicine is expensive and accessible primarily only to the middle and upper classes of most countries.

Where national health insurance, Medicaid, and socialized medicine attempt to resolve the maldistribution of biomedicine in such socialized countries as Sweden and Nigeria, these programs are expensive and susceptible to the political climate. Throughout the rest of the world, biomedicine is available only to that portion of the population that has access to wealth. Even where available for token fees, medical services are often prohibitively expensive when bus fare and absence from work are taken into account.

In Bolivia, as well as in most developing countries, few people have access to biomedicine either because they cannot afford it or because they live in rural areas not served by it. In 1990, the average annual income of a Bolivian factory worker was $500, that of a rural worker, $100. More than half the population of the Department of La Paz are peasant/subsistence farmers. Out of the department's total population of 1,465,078, 52 percent (767,815) live in rural areas with less than 2,000 people per community. These people have little or no access to doctors, nurses, and clinics.

Even in the cities of Bolivia there are inadequate health facilities for the rapidly increasing population. For example, in the peri-urban area of El Alto, Bolivia, with a population of 356,000 in 1990, 5 percent of the families earn from $1 to $15 monthly; 17 percent, from $16 to $30; 23 percent, from $31 to $45; 15 percent, from $46 to $60; 16 percent, from $61 to $100; 10 percent, from $101 to $130; and 14 percent receive payment in specie or have no income (UNITAS 1988:143). For El Alto there is one hospital with thirty beds, seven clinics, thirty-eight doctors, fourteen dentists, thirteen nurses, and sixty-four auxiliary nurses (del Castillo 1983). This is one hospital bed per 12,000 people, one doctor per 9,400 people, one dentist per 25,500 people, and one nurse per 5,500 people. Biomedical coverage in El Alto is about one-tenth that of an industrial country.

In spite of endemic poverty and the paucity of biomedicine, the people of El Alto prefer biomedicine and self-medication to ethnomedicine: 28 percent frequent public health clinics, 25 percent apply self-medication, 21 percent attend private clinics, 16 percent go to social security clinics, 6 percent go to ethnic healers, and 4 percent frequent community health workers and cooperative and church clinics (UNITAS 1988:117). The population of El Alto consists primarily of migrants from rural areas who tend to abandon their traditional medical practices of the past and endeavor to integrate themselves by a dynamic process of "absorption-adoption" of biomedical practices, especially those associated with Western culture (UNITAS 1988:123).

Biomedicine is not readily accessible to rural populations (Phillips 1990:23). In Bolivia, geographical barriers (mountains, rivers, and tropical forests) present obstacles to getting primary health care. In 1980, a doctor refused to go to the remote villages of Province Bautista Saavedra to inoculate the children against various childhood diseases because it was a long and difficult journey. As a

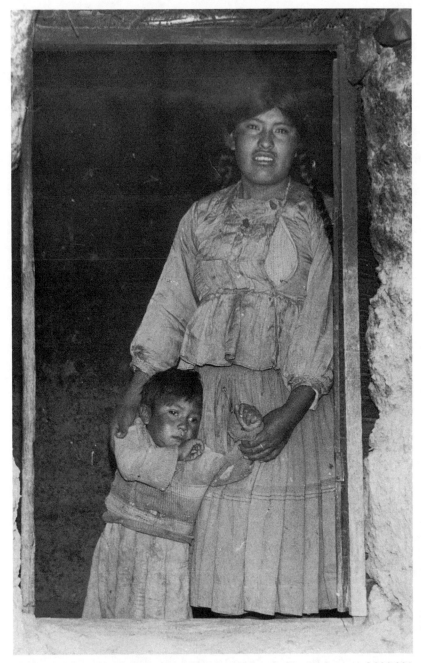

Mother and son in El Alto, a rapidly growing semiurbanized area of 300,000 people without a hospital. Because of the very high incidence of infectious diseases, migrants prefer antibiotics to herbal medicines.

result 200 babies died in a measles epidemic, leaving the population (13,500) of the Kallawaya ethnic group with a depleted generation of infants. In 1990, Kallawaya herbalists themselves provided immunizations for children in these remote communities under the supervision of the doctor in Charazani. Utilization of ethnomedical practitioners thus extended the coverage of biomedicine to communities distant from clinics and otherwise dependent upon the caprices of unpredictable health professionals.

Since the cost of biomedical care is so high that most donor institutions and countries have to continually subsidize the health-care projects, health planners are hesitant to place costly medical services and personnel in areas where the people cannot afford it. The USAID-funded community health-worker program in Montero, Bolivia, is a case in point (Crandon-Malamud 1983). After an investment of $5 million, it was abandoned because neither the United States nor the Bolivian governments were able to continue paying the project workers. Much of the high cost for this project stemmed from the fact that USAID required its projects to buy United States goods even though similar items were much cheaper in Bolivia and Brazil. Another reason for abandoning this project: USAID protested the military dictatorship of President García Meza in the 1980s (Libbet Crandon-Malamud, pers. com. 17 December 1990).

Because health planners do not involve community participation when it comes to purchasing costly medical equipment, it is frequently underutilized in Bolivia and other parts of the world. Many of the refrigerators and birth delivery tables donated by UNICEF to Bolivian clinics sit unused, at least for medical purposes. The cost of these items, including purchase, shipping, and delivery, approaches several thousand dollars per clinic. In the Altiplano, Department of Oruro, aluminum medical cases, costing $300 each, were purchased for auxiliary nurses to use. The cases were little used, at least for health purposes, because the Aymara Indians feared they attracted lightning. The value of these items accrues not to the peasants of Bolivia, but rather to the administrators, merchants, and manufacturers.

Even where modern facilities exist, Bolivian doctors and nurses are often inadequately trained to use them. Bolivian medical schools are closed half of the time and are without residency programs, medical journals, or modern laboratories. Also, since doctors and nurses receive little training in public health or cross-cultural communication, those assigned to peasant communities frequently fail to provide *any* biomedicine for the Aymara- and Quechua-speaking

Indians of Bolivia. Adding to the problem is the preference by the majority of Bolivian doctors and nurses to practice in urban areas. If they cannot work in Bolivian cities, they either migrate to wealthier countries or become politicians. This further reduces the number of doctors and nurses for rural areas.

Inequitable distribution of biomedical personnel, inadequate training of doctors and nurses in public health, insensitivity to and nonutilization of ethnomedicine, and the lack of cross-cultural communication are all reasons why peasants in Bolivia, and in other parts of the developing world, have little or no access to primary health care. These factors better explain the rural health crisis in Bolivia, and they are part of the general situation in developing counties described by George Foster (1977): "There are not now, nor will there be in the foreseeable future, sufficient, fully trained health personnel to meet all health needs."

Unanticipated consequences of primary health care create yet further limitations of biomedicine. Where immunization programs and prenatal care have not been accompanied by development programs and increased agricultural productivity, overpopulation has emerged as a serious health threat. Improving health care for the elderly has prolonged life beyond economic productivity and siphoned scarce medical funds away from children, who have limited status in comparison to the aged. The immediate results provided by antibiotics and steroids have caused peasants to believe unduly in the effects of injections. Many insist upon receiving a shot for whatever malady, and become excessively dependent on drugs. These mistakes could have been avoided had primary health-care workers involved the community in health projects. Brigitte Jordan (1990:114–15) refers to this as the "biomedical colonization of communities."

Politics of Biomedicine

Technological procedures, such as immunization programs, introduction of oral rehydration therapy, and curative measures, are less likely to threaten the interests of the prevailing power structure than are fundamental reforms (Pfleiderer and Bichman 1985). Primary health care, however, focuses primarily on the social, political, and environmental causes of illness (WHO and UNICEF 1978:2). It demands a redistribution of resources and social structural transformations (Heggenhougen 1984; Jordan 1990:114; Navarro 1984). It also stimulates political consciousness and grass-roots political expertise (Werner and Bower 1982).

Peasants in Bolivia, as well as in other parts of the developing world, recognize the curative effects of biomedicine, but they are wary of how biomedicine can be used as a political tool to distinguish races and classes and to create dependency relations with industrial countries (see Gish 1979; Morgan 1987). Throughout the industrialized world, and in many parts of the developing world, biomedical technology determines what is to be taken as authoritative knowledge and, in turn, establishes a particular regime of power (Jordan 1990:115). Biomedicine extends its privileged position, founded on science, to power in economics, politics, and class relations. Its role and power is jealously guarded by laws, medical schools, associations, licensing, and language (medical terminology). Peasants thus view biomedicine as serving the powerful group in a society, in which ordinary people lose autonomy over their own lives (Lock 1987a:131; Zola 1978).

In Bolivia, in the 1950s and 1960s, for example, pharmacists and doctors successfully curtailed the influence of Kallawaya herbalists by disparagement, laws, imprisonment, and denial of licenses. Even though some herbalists had incorporated biomedicine into their therapeutic techniques (Bastien 1987:25–32), doctors and politicians depicted Kallawayas as members of an antiquated Inca healing tradition at best and as cheating witch doctors at worst (Oblitas Poblete 1968). The very success of Kallawaya herbalists and the increasing surplus of doctors, many underemployed, exacerbated the situation.

As a counteroffensive, herbalists use cultural categories to limit the hegemony of doctors; in Bolivia they accuse them of taking blood and fat (Bastien 1985). The Kallawaya of Curva violently resist extraction of blood for testing because they believe its quantity is limited and irreplaceable (Rod Burchard, pers. com. 1982). They commonly stereotype doctors as *kharisiris*, mythological figures who steal fat by inserting tubes into the body. To lose fat is a grave matter for Andeans, who consider it a source of force and energy. Supposed *kharisiris* have been stoned to death, as was the technical assistant of a Japanese physical anthropologist who was collecting blood samples in a village in the Department of Oruro.

In 1985, after I investigated allegations that nurses and doctors in certain communities of the Department of Oruro were *kharisiris*, I found that they were being ostracized from the community for charging too much, not attending to the community's medical needs, or politically aligning themselves with upper-class mestizos. The cultural complex of *kharisiris* functioned as a negative licensing system for community health workers. It was a cultural and political mechanism by which the community participated in health matters.

Even though institutions of biomedicine frequently support class distinctions, Margaret Lock points out that it is not a monolithic organization nor a single systematized form of medical practice and beliefs. She writes:

> At the level of physician-patient interaction, it [biomedicine] represents a perpetual reworking of changing values, new knowledge, and new technology (Gaines and Hahn 1985). It most frequently appears to act as a force for conservatism and, at times, of repression, but since its basic business is the management of suffering and pain, which by its very nature raises questions of ambiguity and paradox, it can also act as a stimulus for the creation of new meanings, and hence social action. (1987a:132)

How doctors and nurses can manage suffering and pain along with ethnomedical practitioners in a context that creates new meanings and social action suitable to peasants is covered in chapter 2.

In sum, class distinctions, racism, and exploitation are frequently part of the biomedical milieu in Bolivia as well as other developing countries. These discriminatory aspects of biomedicine plus the fact that it has been the predominant force in primary health care are the reasons why impoverished peasants are slow to accept it, rather than out of ignorance and cultural differences. Although biomedicine has a history of serving "hegemonic" forms of economic, political, and social institutions, it must begin to serve the poor of the world and promote equitable social institutions. At Alma-Ata the World Health Organization recognized this requirement by emphasizing that ethnic medicine and community participation had to be a part of primary health care. The challenge to international health is to remove biomedicine from its hegemonic contexts; to adapt it to cultural, economic, political, and social realities of peoples of the developing world; and to integrate it with ethnomedicine. Primary health care can do this by emphasizing community participation, by utilizing native resources and personnel, and by employing ethnomedicine.

2

Quack Doctors, Superstition, and Witchcraft

WITH HENRI MIGALA

When it comes to ethnomedicine, educated Bolivians, especially doctors, refer to its practitioners as "quack doctors," somehow acquainting them with the traveling medicine men at the turn of the century who were hawking snake oil. The implication is that there are "real doctors" and "phony doctors." Ethnomedical practitioners are also accused of observing superstitions and engaging in witchcraft. After the Spanish conquest of Central and South America, ethnomedical practitioners were forbidden to function as such because their curing techniques were considered heretical. Around the middle of this century, doctors and pharmacists in Bolivia pressured the Bolivian legislature to outlaw ethnomedical practices by requiring licensing. Although a few noted middle-class herbalists obtained licenses, others were unable to and were jailed.

Scholars and doctors may have objections directed toward ethnomedicine, but there are ample reasons for including ethnomedical practitioners in health care. Joseph Bastien began realizing the importance of ethnomedical practitioners in 1966 when he worked as a Maryknoll priest and supervised a primary health clinic in Peñas, Bolivia. Amazed at the success of penicillin shots, Bastien bought vials by the hundreds and injected numerous peasants, curing them rapidly of skin and other bacterial diseases. Weekly, a Spanish doctor visited the clinic to treat serious illnesses. Although Bastien was satisfied with the success of the injections, he was equally frustrated with his inability to treat many illnesses.

The significance of herbalists to Andean health was brought home to Bastien on one memorable occasion. Juan Cadena arrived at the clinic with a dislocated shoulder bone. Juan asked Bastien to drive him to the doctor in La Paz, a journey of an hour and half by jeep, but Bastien was unable to because his jeep was not running. Bastien was deeply concerned, but Cadena said that it was alright and that he would find a *qollasiri* (curer). The next morning Cadena appeared at the rectory door with his shoulder in place. He said that a *qollasiri* had placed compresses of frog skins on his shoulder, given him an infusion made from some strong herbs to drink, and later massaged the shoulder back in place.

In rural areas such as Peñas and other parts of the developing world, peasants rely on ethnomedicine because it is affordable, convenient, and culturally familiar; and ethnomedical practitioners are readily accessible. (For an annotated bibliography on traditional medicine, see Harrison and Cosminsky 1976 and Cosminsky and Harrison 1984.) The World Health Organization describes ethnomedicine as the sum total of all the knowledge and practices, whether explicable or not, used in diagnosis, prevention, and elimination of physical, mental, or social imbalances of a given ethnic group. Ethnomedicine relies primarily on practical experience and observation handed down from one generation to the next.

People transmit ethnomedical systems by oral and written traditions. Ayurvedic medicine in India and the Hippocratic-Galenic humoral theory that spread from Greece, Italy, Arabia, and Spain to Latin America are two ancient traditions transmitted in writing over a thousand years. These were great traditions maintained by the literati and supported by the ruling classes. Highly sophisticated, they perdure and are popular among peoples in Africa, China, India, and Latin America, even where biomedicine was introduced long ago (see Leslie 1976 and Kleinman 1980).

Lesser ethnomedical traditions are usually oral traditions varying with the narrator, community, and experiences of the time. Often referred to as folk healing, these types of medical traditions are embedded in practical experience learned and communicated by indigenous healers. Dependent on community ideology, folk healing traditions are dynamic, living traditions that do not adapt well to standardization, regulation, and institutionalization—one reason why folk healers do not want to be governed by the dominant medical establishment.

Both greater and lesser medical traditions are available in Bolivia: the Hippocratic-Galenic humoral theory of the balance of hot, cold, wet, and dry; the Western biomedical theory of destroying germs and classifying diseases; and the Andean topographic-hydraulic theory of the centripetal and centrifugal flow of fluids between the body and the environment (Bastien 1985). These three systems are coterminous with many distinct and variable folk traditions at community and tribal levels, especially those of the Amazon. There is an evolving syncretic ethnomedical system that includes elements from these two traditions. Bolivians thus have the advantage of choosing from many alternative medical traditions that provide many resources for health and more possibilities for primary health care. Meeting the criteria of the World Health Organization (1977:89), Bolivian ethnomedical practitioners are recognized by their community as competent to provide health care using vegetable, animal, and mineral substances and certain other methods based on social, cultural, and religious practices as well as on the knowledge, attitudes, values, and beliefs that are prevalent in the community regarding physical, mental, and social well-being and the causation of disease and diseasability.

Neumann and Lauro (1982) categorize ethnomedical practitioners as spiritual or magico-religious healers (such as diviners, shamans, *espiritistas,* and ritualists); herbalists (such as herbal vendors and ethnopharmacologists); manipulators (such as bonesetters, hydrotherapists, masseurs, and "suckers"); and birth attendants (such as midwives and traditional birth attendants). Some ethnomedical practitioners in Bolivia perform functions of all four categories and some do not fit into any of these categories. Some, such as herbalists, midwives, bonesetters, and masseurs, follow empirical methods and are more acceptable to biomedical practitioners than diviners, ritualists, shamans, sorcerers, and witches, who deal with extraordinary reality. Yet the latter greatly influence illness and health in the community.

In the village of Qaqachaka in the 1980s the *wayt'iri* (shaman) and auxiliary nurse competed with each other for medical control of the village. The nurse discredited the shaman as a fraud and his magic as nonsense; the shaman attacked the nurse's legitimacy by telling the villagers that the *sajjra* (devil) dwelt beneath the clinic and influenced the nurse's medical practice. Qaqachakans avoided the clinic and shunned the nurse until he collaborated more with the shaman. The role of magic, especially black, has little acceptance in biomedicine, with its ethics based on preservation of life; but in many cultures, sorcery and witchcraft play a disciplinary role in the community and are prophylactics against greater maladies.

The World Health Organization endorses the use of ethnomedical practitioners in national health programs for several reasons. Following independence from colonial rule in the 1950s and 1960s, many countries assumed a national identity associated with a conception of their native heritage, and ethnomedicine provided a rich source for establishing identity, more so than biomedicine with its colonial heritage. In addition, WHO's endorsement recognized that developing countries have minimal economic resources with which to extend health care to rural people and that ethnomedicine provided an available and low-cost resource (Akerele 1983).

In the opinion of the World Health Organization (1978), ethnomedical practitioners have become stagnated by not exploiting the rapid discoveries of science and technology. As a critic, Velimirovic (1990:52) points out that ethnomedicine has not helped indigenous people against cholera and other enteric infections, such as sleeping sickness, yellow fever, leprosy, schistosomiasis, trachoma, onchocercosis, malaria, and tuberculosis, that have decimated people. He adds that it has not lowered death rates, still averaging 93 per 1,000 births. Infant mortality rates are as high as 200 per 1,000 in some developing countries (Velimirovic 1990:52). However, he overlooks the fact that the slow rate of change among ethnomedical practitioners is characteristic of societies not yet immersed in industrialization. Once doctors collaborate with ethnomedical practitioners, the latter more readily accept biomedical discoveries. Neither can ethnomedical practitioners be blamed for not lowering disease and death rates that are affected more by economic, political, and social factors than by the inadequacy of ethnomedicine. Poverty brought about by the exploitation of peasants brings starvation and malnutrition, which contribute greatly to high infant mortality rates. Malaria and tuberculosis were introduced after the conquest in Latin America, and ethnomedical practitioners have not yet evolved cures for these "foreign" diseases. Malaria is a behavioral-driven disease in that garbage and stagnant sewage contribute greatly to its spread. Even though in Bangladesh, for example, biomedicine eradicated malaria by insecticides fifteen years ago, it is now prevalent in endemic numbers because of persistent problems with sewage and drainage as well as mosquitos resistant to DDT and discontinued spraying. The fact that the very hegemonic system promoting biomedicine is responsible for increases in malnutrition, infant mortality, and morbidity in the last century has its unmistakable effects on presently marginalized populations.

By emphasizing ethnomedicine, directors of WHO were trying to provide a balance in heavily biomedically dominated international health systems. Citing the shortcomings of ethnomedicine, the World Health report (1978) unequivocally concludes with the following:

> Traditional medicine has been shown to have intrinsic utility, it should be promoted, and its potential developed for the wider use and benefit of mankind. It is already the people's own health care

system and is well accepted by them. It has certain advantages over imported systems of medicine in any setting because, as an integral part of the people's culture, it is particularly effective in solving certain cultural health problems. It has and does contribute to scientific and universal medicine.

Since 1978 this directive has been little followed by international health agencies except for the United States Agency for International Development (USAID). Efforts to integrate ethnomedicine with biomedicine in primary health care are minimal throughout the world (Bourne 1987).) An exception is Bolivia where biomedical and ethnomedical practitioners are beginning to collaborate in primary health care. Without doing so, biomedicine and primary health care cannot meet their goals (Chabot 1984; *The Economist* 1985; Mull 1990; Jordan 1990).

Objections to the Use of Indigenous Healers

Advocates of the biomedical paradigm complain that ethnomedicine is not scientific and that ethnomedical practitioners have not accepted biomedical practices. For these reasons, and others, many people oppose ethnomedicine (see Slikkerveer 1982). Before the Alma-Ata conference, when the developed world was less enthusiastic about the role of folk healers in health planning, George Foster (1977:531–34) wrote that the number of traditional healers would decrease in the face of increasingly available biomedical services, and would not constitute an adequate manpower reservoir to assist in an appropriate health service for developing countries. He added that some traditional remedies are dangerous and that these treatments could delay referral to medical doctors, resulting in a routine treatment such as an appendectomy becoming vastly more complicated. Harrison (1974–75:12) found that most government personnel in Nigeria doubted the value of folk healers because the healers were "superstitious," secretive, and difficult to evaluate and to train. Even today, some fifteen years later, after such ideas have long been discredited by international health professionals as well as encoded in WHO policy (WHO and UNICEF 1978), government personnel, doctors, and nurses in most countries are still skeptical of the value of folk healers.

Contributing to this skepticism are the views of developing countries' policy makers and health administrators who believe the incorporation of ethnomedical practitioners to be "second class medicine" (Pillsbury 1979:13–14). This attitude is a consequence of the colonial legacy in which Western biomedicine went to Asia, Africa, and Latin America to serve the needs of European and American colonizers and entrepreneurs. In newly independent nations, laws and regulations have been passed making indigenous practitioners, including midwives, "illegal." After upwardly mobile natives became educated in schools dominated by European thought, they psychologically distanced themselves from ethnic ways, including their own healing traditions.

In 1985, Joseph Bastien presented a talk on the Kallawaya herbal tradition to a group of mestizo physicians at the general hospital in Oruro, Bolivia. One doctor vehemently protested against the peasants using this medicine and, shouting expletives, stormed out of the room. The next day, another surgeon apologized for his behavior and explained that this doctor's mother was an important *chiflera* (herbal vendor) in Oruro. Cultural hegemony can explain his attempt to disassociate himself from his family tradition in that he was relatively insecure in his new role as an empirically trained doctor and feared that he would be linked with "magical" practices.

Another biomedical objection to the practice of ethnomedicine is that it can be potentially dangerous. Some examples are cautery or bleeding to expel "bad blood" (Tunisia); application of cow-dung ash, a likely carrier of tetanus bacteria, to dry up the umbilical cord (South Asia); sweeping with a broom the lower abdominal area of a woman's body, following delivery, to remove the placenta (Haiti); and clitoredectomy with rudimentary instruments, accompanied by a high incidence of AIDS (Africa).

These critics overlook the fact that both ethnomedicine and biomedicine adopt practices that are worthless. When biomedical intervention actually injures a person's health, it is viewed as being iatrogenic. Biomedicine no less than any other medical approach needs continual reevaluation to assess its therapeutic effects. Furthermore, ethnomedicine includes many beneficial practices discounted in biomedicine. They contribute to the self-healing process because of secondary effects—meaning, group acceptance, catharsis, and spirituality—far more so than biomedicine can. And they have important tertiary effects upon the community, environment, and religion. The elaborate curing rituals of Kallawaya diviners bring participants together from three different farming and herding zones to share resources and to symbolically reiterate the unity of resource exchange (Bastien 1978).

Thus, health educators would best serve their populations if they incorporated indigenous practitioners into the medical system and, at the same time, encouraged the modification of certain practices and beliefs about disease causation. Kallawaya herbalists have always sought to adopt new treatments through observation and practice, and would be pleased to learn that syphilis is not caused by urinating in the wind or the fire, that tuberculosis is not the result of indulging in intercourse with a fever, that blindness is not caused by the wrath of God, that leprosy is not caused by touching a person of lower caste, and that diarrhea is not caused by fright (see Velimirovic 1990:533). Few, if any, ethnomedical practitioners continue practices they discover are harmful to the person's health.

Once Bolivian doctors and nurses are shown the value and significance of ethnomedicine, be it hermeneutical, biological, psychological, or cultural, they often accept it with enthusiasm. They recognize, in spite of their upward social mobility, the harm done to them and their culture by the legacy of colonialism and the cultural hegemony of neocolonialism. If some value is attached to Aymara ethnomedicine, mestizo doctors and nurses will no longer need to oppose it. Remaining Aymara, they can continue their upward mobility, have access to more clientele, and gain prestige among varying classes of people.

Prejudice against alternative medical traditions is not a one-way street. In the present postcolonial period, natives in certain African countries are being denied biomedicine by the advocacy of a rigid form of ethnomedical traditionalism. Philip Singer (1977:3) has discussed how the hegemony of the colonialists has been supplanted by that of native black rulers. Except among the rulers themselves, this new colonialism does not provide the rural masses with biomedicine, promoting ethnomedicine instead. Such promotion symbolically supports dictatorial regimes in the name of an ethnically defined nationalism (see Last 1986), but it leads to curious results. Chief Lambo of the Yoruba in Nigeria, for example, refers to the following technique as a "wonder in nature." A Yoruba man becomes jealous of his wife because she refuses to have sex with the frequency he demands. He consults a medicine man, who has the woman pass over a knotted string. This tightens the vagina so that no penis may enter. She is now believed to be a "werewolf." When the man wishes to "redeem" the woman, he unties the knot. As Singer (1977:3) points out: "Traditionalism is as much a 'force' and 'social process' as is colonialism. Because it is 'traditional' does not make it 'better' or anti-colonial."

Faced with this option, health planners frequently object that they are unable to evaluate the quality of care provided by ethnomedical practitioners because there is usually no formal system of regulation or licensure that planners and administrators can utilize to distinguish competent from incompetent practitioners (Nchinda 1976; Pillsbury 1979:16). When ethnomedical practitioners are licensed or attain positions of importance within the biomedical establishment, they frequently compromise ethnomedical practices to meet biomedical standards, such as Mario Salcedo, a licensed Kallawaya herbalist who assumes a formal manner like a medical doctor to gain approval. Their association with biomedical practitioners or institutions often seriously hampers their communication and effectiveness with rural peoples (Alvarado 1978:20). Maria Chuca, a midwife in the Department of Potosí, Bolivia, lost her clientele in the community of Ara after she adopted certain biomedical practices taught in a training course for midwives. Resisting changes, villagers selected a midwife who followed exclusively traditional practices.

If folk healers are evaluated by the rules of the bureaucratic health establishment, they lose their cultural flexibility. Folk medicine, like folk music, plays an integral part in ordinary peasants' lives. It reflects people's concerns, beliefs, and needs.

Incompetence is, of course, also a problem among doctors and nurses, but it can presumably be detected by formal systems of regulation and licensure. In contrast to such formal regulative processes, however, which require adherence to rules, tests, and supervision, folk practitioners are evaluated by the community according to how well they perform the role expected of them. The competence of these practitioners can be evaluated in terms of objectives and standards unique to the medical system, whether it be physiological improvement, spiritual awareness, community solidarity, alliance with ancestors, restoration of something lost, or removal of some object. Would it be fair to discredit a medical doctor for not properly diagnosing a patient with demonic possession when this is not within his or her field? Communities do have criteria for recognizing competent medical practitioners that include accessibility, availability, acceptability, dependability, and effectiveness (Nchinda 1976; Phillips 1990:63–102; Pillsbury 1979:16).

The Kallawaya, for example, are world-famous herbalists, and in the village of Chajaya there are more than thirty of them. The community recognizes varying ranks of herbal skills as clearly as baseball fans know who the hitters are. Competence is recognizable in practice, and peasants frugal with their limited resources find out "through the grapevine" who the best healers are. Although some ethnomedical practitioners are "incompetent" according to biomedical standards, they are known, respected, and trainable. The value of ethnomedical practitioners and their incorporation into biomedical systems has become widely accepted since the advocacy of WHO in 1978, but the high cost of training folk healers, the reluctance of the health bureaucracy to accept them, and the general decline of folk medicine have discouraged such incorporation. Doctors and nurses believe that practitioners of ethnomedicine need to be educated and regulated before they can participate in primary health care. Granted that both biomedical and ethnomedical practitioners need to understand each other's methods, refer patients, and share common objectives, it is essential to recognize that ethnic medicine is valuable on its own folk terms and becomes less valuable once it's regulated, licensed, and bureaucratized, as Margaret Lock (1987:7–9) and Libbet Crandon-Malamud (pers. com. 1990) have pointed out. Nonetheless, ethnomedical practitioners need to be legally accepted as health practitioners by national governments and ministries of health and provided with the freedom to practice. The objective of an integrated health program is to grant them this legal and professional autonomy as well as to educate them in abandoning worthless practices and to teach people about public health measures.

Advantages of Ethnomedical Practitioners

The efforts to incorporate ethnomedical and biomedical practices are worthwhile because the dual approach leaves nothing missing. In this age of "Save the Earth," ethnomedical practitioners use adaptive strategies and folk traditions that are living and dynamic systems subject to change in response to environment and community, providing examples of biocultural integration. Bolivian as well as other Andean medical systems provide a myriad of adaptive strategies to some of the most variable environmental zones of the world, from the tropical Amazon to the high sierras.

Another advantage is that ethnomedical practitioners are a readily available resource. A basic premise of humanistic development, what is considered appropriate technology is the use of native resources and personnel whenever possible. This approach to development attempts to minimize peoples' dependence on "outsiders" and costly resources and technology (Jordan 1990). One problem with health development agencies is that by exporting expensive technological medical systems they make the inhabitants of developing countries too dependent on the wealthier donor countries. In Bolivia, for example, administrators of international health projects and ministries of health purchase expensive drugs and then pressure health workers to sell these to repay the debt. The need for income is so urgent in health projects that doctors and nurses are encouraged to sell more pharmaceuticals than perhaps required, which has made some peasants drug dependent. In 1984, a director of UNICEF tried to convince Gregory Rake, director of Project Concern, to become involved in the distribution of several million overstocked pharmaceuticals in Bolivian warehouses that needed to be sold before their effective dates expired. Rake refused partially because he stocks medicinal plants in the clinics that he supervises. The successful marketing of pharmaceuticals has made some peasants so dependent on injections that they complain if they are not given one at each office visit. Doctors and nurses often use the same syringe for numerous vaccinations, frequently without sterilizing it, in order to increase their income, or subsidize the project, or economize if not enough syringes have been supplied. In a country as rich as Bolivia in plants and herbal knowledge, this dependency on synthetic drugs could be lessened by utilizing herbalists and medicinal plants.

Investment in indigenous practitioners holds down costs significantly and provides an affordable way for peasants to receive health care. They far outnumber biomedical practitioners, as in Swaziland where there is one ethnomedical healer (not including traditional birth attendants) per 110 population compared to about one physician per 10,000 population (Green 1985:283). In Bolivia there is at least one midwife, shaman, and herbalist for every rural community with a population ranging from 200 to 1,000 people compared to about one physician per 7,000 in population. Trained by experience, these practitioners are part of the community they serve and readily available, and they adjust their fees according to the income of the peasants. Most important, ethnomedicine and its practitioners provide an available resource that involves community participation and depends less on government politics, foreign aid, and a wealthier nation's generosity, which sometimes has strings attached.

Social and Cultural Methods of Healing

Economics and availability provide strong reasons for utilizing ethnomedical practitioners, but even stronger reasons are that they provide therapies that deal with social and cultural aspects of illnesses. Traditional healers often involve the entire family as well as the community in the process of diagnosis and treatment. Ethnomedicine begins at the household level, where family members possess a great deal of information bearing on the diagnosis and treatment of common symptoms. The family not only provides emotional support to patients but also motivates them to follow the prescribed treatment. Beyond the family there exists a whole range of specialists, herbalists, diviners, bonesetters and accredited experts on different conditions, such as psychiatric illness and women's and children's ailments. By diagnosing the cause of disease and prescribing corrective measures, ethnomedical healers exert social control on the family and community. *Limpu*, a culturally defined fatal illness in Bolivia, moves from patient to patient—a public health hazard according to Bolivian perceptions. If the healer is from Ancoraimes, he or she has a real interest in preventing the spread of this disease and in the patients' health (Crandon-Malamud 1987:465).

Frequently, illnesses are related to social relationships, which indigenous practitioners address. The people of Challapata, for example, eighty kilometers south of Oruro, associate *susto* (loss of animating fluid) and depression with lack of love, and they cure these ailments by group ritual—a form of supportive therapy. They are also more concerned about liver ailments than tuberculosis because liver trouble leads to anger, which disrupts the family. For Andeans in general, sicknesses are considered serious if they affect social relations. They define being sick as when someone is unable to work. Moreover, they believe that ill people should be cured in the home with the family participating. The father gathers medicinal plants, the mother prepares special meals, and siblings and cousins pray. They sit beside the sick person during the night and console him or her during the day. They dislike hospitals with their dreaded antiseptic smells and white, sterile walls. (White is often associated with the death and burial of babies by Andeans.) In Qaqachaka, 140 kilometers south of Oruro, Bastien wanted to transport a dying man with tuberculosis to the hospital in Challapata, but the Indians refused, saying that he would die in the hospital if he was taken from his family and home (Bastien 1987).

Kallawaya herbalists recognize the importance of family therapy and make house calls. One advantage traveling Kallawayas have always had over their sedentary colleagues was the ability to heal rural Andeans in their villages and homes. Since many Andeans live in hamlets far away from clinics, transporting sick people in the backs of crowded trucks often worsens their conditions. Home is the

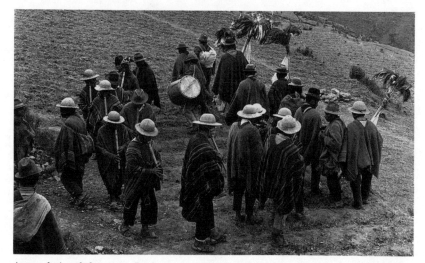

Annual ritual dance to Pachamama (Mother Earth) by Kallawayas of Kaata so the earth will provide them with nutrients to stay healthy. The dancers move centripetally, symbolizing returning to the center of the earth, then centrifugally, symbolizing their understanding of fluids entering the body, concentrating, and dispersing to parts of the body—a metaphor of health and the body.

preferred site for curing because of its proximity to environmental and symbolic causes of illnesses. For Andeans of the Bolivian Altiplano, ruptures in their relationships with animals, plants, and land are attributable as causes of sicknesses (see Bastien 1987).

As in Bolivia, ethnomedical practitioners throughout the world are deeply involved in the maintenance of social order and in preserving cultural institutions (see Crandon-Malamud 1983b). They help the patient live at peace with his or her family, clan, village, tribe, and him- or herself. Such healers have a broader social role to play and are more community-oriented than the typical biomedical clinician. Ethnomedical practitioners are not limited to drugs or herbs, frequently using spiritual rituals and the regulation of diet and behavior. Being from the community, ethnomedical healers can also act as social engineers for primary health care (Maclean and Bannerman 1982:1815).

Ethnomedical practitioners' biggest asset is that they deal with etiological factors communicated by symbolic and cultural expressions as well as by biological and psychological symptoms to classify illness as a biocultural phenomenon. Nurses and doctors, on the other hand, focus primarily on biological features of the complaint to classify an illness according to biomedical science. Etiologically, ethnomedical practitioners are more concerned with how the symptoms relate to natural, supernatural, ritual, psychological, physiological, and social factors. They address the culturally shaped multiplicity of meanings understood by sick people and their relatives (see B. Good 1977:25–28; Van Schaik 1989:15–28; and A. Young 1982:257–85).

Once they have identified the causes in popular terms, healers use therapeutic devices familiar to the patient, including foods and drinks, taboos and beliefs, and prayers and rituals. Patients feel at home with these therapies, providing a sense of control and involvement.

To illustrate this: while Joseph Bastien was doing fieldwork in Kaata, Bolivia, he and other members of Marcelino Yanahuaya's family became sick, so they invited Rosinta Garcia, a *curandera*, from the neighboring village to perform a misfortune ritual (Bastien 1978, 1980). Well after midnight, Rosinta, in order to divine the cause of the illness, used a guinea pig that had been placed on her forehead. She exposed its viscera with her fingernails and poured its blood into a cup with wine, eggs, and corn. After removing the rib cage, she examined the protrusion in the front, which formed a small half-moon. She then spotted two incisions, which she said were two mouths (*simikuna*). Enemies were bewitching Bastien and the family members, she explained, and Marcelino identified one mouth as that of Dominga Air. Dominga had become impoverished following the death of her husband, Mariano Yanahuaya. Twenty years earlier, Mariano, Marcelino's classificatory brother, had usurped Marcelino's land, and Marcelino said that Dominga's blindness and poverty were the punishment from his ancestors. In fact, Dominga had accused Marcelino of soliciting a sorceress to send these misfortunes. When two hostile Andean families suffer calamities, an exchange of sorcery is suspected.

Sorcery causes sickness and has to be removed, so Rosinta proceeded to dispel it. She prepared a meal for the river, which symbolizes the removal of evil. She laid a rat at the head of a ritual cloth and sorted out twenty wads of dark llama wool. Slivers of pig fat were put on coca leaves and placed on the wads as she declared that this was the sickness being dispelled. She rubbed the participants' bodies with the wads and placed others in the crops, weavings, the kitchen, sleeping room, and dispensary. The sheep, horse, and burro corrals were each given two wads. After the wads had drawn the evil forces from the associated objects, they were placed beneath the hats or headbands worn by participants and inside their sandals next to their feet to be taken to the river.

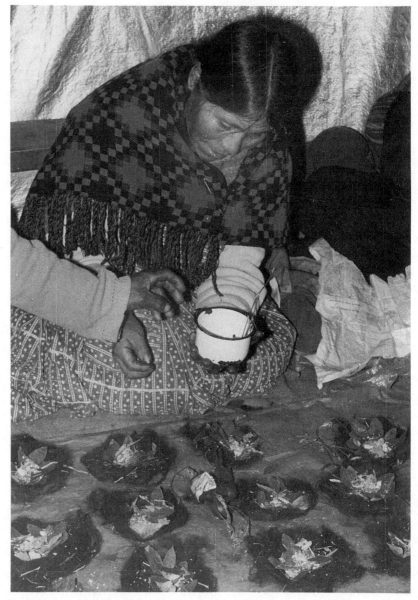

Rosinta Garcia performing a misfortune ritual in Kaata to cure Erminia Yana-huaya. Erminia recovered for several months, but eventually died of septice-mia. She was also treated by medical doctors.

Participants stumbled along in the dark, Marcelino at the front and Rosinta at the end. They arrived at the Kunochayuh river and climbed up to a cave alongside it. They knelt facing the river's descent. Rosinta threw the yolk and white from a chicken egg into the waters and then removed the black wads from the hats and sandals as well as from the women's headbands. As she broke the headbands, she also broke the wool threads around the participants' hands and feet. She put the black wads into an old coca cloth with the guinea pig, rat, coca quids, cigarette butts, and ashes. Everyone looked away as Rosinta flung the cloth into the river, saying, *"Puriy-* chej chijekuna!" ("Begone misfortunes!").

Rosinta revealed that the sickness was related to ancestors, ancestral land, backbiting, loss of land, and bodily ailments. She then helped the participants dispel their sicknesses by projecting them into wads and throwing them into the river. She provided a continuity within the patients' experiences of bodily disintegration. Because of Rosinta and this ritual, the participants felt that they had control over the sicknesses. The psychological value was that patients visualized the misfortunes and were able to manipulate them by symbolic means that they believed in. This affected the dispositions and immune systems of patients. Indeed, after the ritual, participants improved in health.

This case illustrates the value of ethnomedical practitioners as providing a discourse of cultural significance beyond any empirical effects of treatment. Moreover, they offer patients social and cultural continuity at times when diseases have disintegrating effects on their bodies.

Admittedly, Rosinta provided negligible permanent cures for the virulent disease agents causing respiratory problems for the Yanahuayas. The fact that ethnomedical practitioners often do not have cures for many disease agents is reason for their being integrated with biomedical practitioners.

Integration of Biomedical
and Ethnomedical Practitioners

Throughout the world, successful efforts to improve rural health have been made in the last twenty years by incorporating midwives and other ethnomedical practitioners into primary health care. Development efforts have encouraged midwives to practice hygiene and refer difficult cases to government health services. Health-development personnel have recognized that ethnomedical healers can contribute to the treatment of mental illness because patient expectation is an important element in therapy (Garrison 1974, 1977; Ruiz and Langrod 1976). Furthermore, they recognize that the cost of replacing shamans with medically trained psychiatrists would be prohibitive. Village shamans often alleviate those mental illnesses not caused by organic dysfunction. Torrey (1973:119) claims that "witch doctors" get about the same therapeutic results as psychiatrists do. Imagine what the cost would be to have psychiatrists practicing across the Bolivian Altiplano.

The therapist-spiritist training project in Puerto Rico, a project that successfully integrated ethnomedical healing practices with mental-health services, is a case in point (Koss 1980:255–66). This project endeavored to establish a forum for the meaningful exchange of information between the two healing systems (spiritism and community mental health), to offer training to both systems, and to develop new psychotherapeutic approaches from a synthesis of the most relevant and effective healing techniques in each system. Results were less than planned, but one important outcome was a referral unit in which referrals by therapists to known spiritists can be monitored as well as those by spiritists to particular units, and therapists in the mental health center can continue to include treatment by the referring spiritist. An important change occurred among participating spiritists in that they gradually coalesced into a collaborative group, whereas previously they were divisive and competitive as healers associated with different centers and with distinct beliefs within the spiritist movement. For example, seven spiritists became actively involved in the activities and services of the mental-health center.

These values of ethnomedicine and its practitioners as well as the limitations of Western biomedicine are strong arguments for an integrated primary health-care system which takes from each tradition those elements that best satisfy the needs of a particular community. The realities of persistent poverty and inadequate resources in less developed countries seem lost on those planners reluctant to consider ethnomedical practitioners as a valuable resource, especially for serving hard-to-reach populations. Unfortunately, biomedicine has become so highly specialized that many of its professionals, regardless of nationality, develop a "trained incapacity" to consider the holistic sociocultural context in which health care is sought, stressing instead sophisticated technology and clinical procedure (Pillsbury 1979:13–14).

Another impediment in the integration of ethnomedicine with biomedicine is the legal status of ethnomedical practitioners. National codes of law, usually Western-oriented legacies of colonialism, are limited in their capability of expressing indigenous medical conceptions. Establishing ethnomedical legitimacy by modern legal codes is impeded by the inability of most state laws to legally define witchcraft, spirits and magic, divination, and ritual curing. Bibeau (1982:1843–49) concludes for Zaire that if health planners really want to maintain the specific characteristics of ethnomedicine, they have only two solutions: either to declare this medicine illegal, a solution that is unacceptable because it is in complete contradiction to people's actual way of life, or to legalize it and, at the same time, give the healers, through their associations, the main power of selection and control of their activities. As already discussed for Bolivia, if ethnomedical practitioners are legalized, they should not be subjected to licensing and control by members of the dominant medical establishment.

Yet another impediment is patient referral. Patients frequently consult both biomedical and ethnomedical practitioners for the same illness: sometimes in sequence, sometimes concurrently. Throughout the developing world, physicians complain that their patients come to the hospital with advanced stages of disease after their consultations with local healers have failed to cure them (see Yoder 1982:1851–57).

Patients' choice of medical practitioners is a point in question that needs research in each country. What factors determine the kind of health care sought? Near Lake Titicaca in Ancoraimes, Bolivia, medical choice is based not on medical efficacy but on political concerns, as Libbet Crandon-Malamud (1991) points out. Through the primary resource of medicine, people have access to secondary resources, the principal one being social mobility. Tracing Ancoraimes's history and formation of social class in the first half of the twentieth century, Libbet exposes precisely what the secondary resources are, why they exist, and how medical theory has molded and been molded by history. The medical systems themselves are highly fluid, changing through the incremental uses, choices, and opinions of all the individuals seeking health care. People of Ancoraimes resort equally to both indigenous and cosmopolitan medicine.

The fact that Bolivians and peoples of other developing countries resort equally to ethno- and biomedicine provides a basis for instituting a system of mutual referral. Mutual referral depends entirely on the willingness of practitioners to accept "alternative" kinds of treatment as having some merit. One step toward ascertaining merit is to have both kinds of practitioners observe each other's practice. Given the history of mutual ignorance and distrust, plus a claim to exclusive knowledge and "truth" in certain domains, persuading them to observe other kinds of treatment in an unfamiliar setting is difficult. Yet all practitioners are interested in therapy, and many realize their limitations. In Zaire, doctors and nurses followed these stages: first they researched patients' choices of alternative therapies and ethnomedical practitioners' case loads, then they observed "alternative" kinds of treatment, and finally they discussed methods of referral (Yoder 1982:1855–56). In Bolivia, a successful method of referral has been to have integrated clinics in which both ethnomedical and biomedical personnel practice together.

Referral of patients is an indicator of how well the health system is functioning. If doctors fear that they will lose patients, they will not refer them to other practitioners. When ethnomedical practitioners refer patients to doctors, they risk being dismissed and losing the income. For referral to work, it has to be mutual: both parties have to get something out of the exchange. Integration of ethnomedical practioners into the health system is essential to make a system of mutual referral work, but what is meant by integration?

Theories of Integration

Cross-cultural research provides theories of integration of pluralistic medical systems. In India, the dynamics of the relationship between ethno- and biomedicine are evident in three viewpoints: naive scientistic, agnostic anthropological, and political structuralist (Jeffery 1982:1835–41). Predominately preached by British doctors during the colonial epoch and common among Indian doctors today, the naive scientistic view assumes that ethnomedical systems are steadily giving ground to the onward march of science, although the Indian doctors express guarded sympathy and support for the relevance of ethnomedicine. The agnostic-anthropological viewpoint is presented by Charles Leslie (1976:10) in describing Asian medical systems as "coexisting normative institutions." This viewpoint assumes that cultural processes of change are not simply unidirectional (with ethnomedicine being affected by biomedicine and not vice versa) but multidirectional, with no predictions of necessary future patterns. The political-structuralist viewpoint contends that biomedicine will absorb ethnomedicine, not because of scientific superiority but because it is more closely linked to class interests of the political leadership of India (Banerji 1978; Frankenberg 1978).

Ethnomedicine in India is essentially marginalized, with many of its practitioners working part-time, dealing with a limited range of ailments, drawing heavily on biomedical pharmacopoeia, and perceiving biomedicine as superior (Jeffery 1982:1840). Government policy, particularly in terms of employment and expenditure, reinforces this trend. Nonetheless, ethnomedicine is gaining greater respect with the aid of its practitioners in getting people to register health cards and with the recognition of indigenous contributions by international agencies, especially in regard to community health-worker projects. Unfortunately in India and other places, woman healers are being marginalized and excluded from positions of influence.

Health policy makers are looking for ways to incorporate ethnomedicine into the national health policy. The challenge is to do this and avoid a synchretism wherein either ethnomedical practitioners practice aspects of scientific medicine without the appropriate training or biomedical practitioners adopt aspects of ethnomedicine out of context. Yet, once ethnomedical practitioners are integrated with biomedical practitioners, changes will occur.

Scholars differ as to the appropriate extent of integration and the role of ethnomedical practitioners. Their views can be categorized as either autonomous or syncretic. Advocating autonomy, Alvarado (1978:20) writes that meaningful cooperation between bio- and ethnomedical practitioners should be based on complete autonomy for each and that the proper role of the ethnomedical practitioner should be one of a consultant, independent of financial or other ties to the attending physician. Patients and their families select with advice from a doctor an acceptable ethnomedical practitioner, but the physician is not held responsible if the ethnomedical treatment is unsuccessful. This way the doctor can suggest ethnomedical practitioners who are experienced in treating the physical symptoms expressed by the patient. It requires that the doctor be knowledgeable about ethnomedicine, its contributions to biomedicine, and the varying skills of ethnomedical practitioners.

The favorable aspects of autonomy are that both medicines are seen as components of a competitive and complementary relationship, that they can maintain an independence, and that ethnomedicine is not controlled by the bureaucratic medical establishment (see Leslie 1980). The unfavorable aspects are that autonomous systems frequently result in low levels of integration and communication between practitioners of biomedicine and ethnomedicine. This is undesirable for a comprehensive and coordinated rural health program. Moreover, without referrals, both practitioners tend to compete with one another for the limited amount of medical dollars.

A modified version of the autonomy model is proposed wherein ethnomedical practitioners are allowed their independence but are provided with training programs to enhance their skills as well as to remove maladaptive practices, such as educating midwives to use sterile procedures or advising herbalists about the toxicity of some plants. Modification implies that ethnomedical practitioners are not completely left alone to fend for themselves within a political economy in which they are at a disadvantage, but rather that they are trained to be more competitive, provided with structures to protect their position within this economy, and integrated into health projects (see Morgan 1987:144). Autonomy is modified through bilateral communication, between biomedical and ethnomedical practitioners, of information that is beneficial to both without the fear of losing clientele.

Project Concern employed this model in Oruro, Bolivia, by training herbalists and midwives in more salubrious practices and helping them establish associations independent of the doctors and nurses. Project Concern also sponsored a convocation of herbalists in Bolivia in July 1985 to exchange information about medicinal plants. By 1990, however, doctors and nurses had discontinued efforts at integrating ethnomedicine because project directors did not promote it, but associations of ethnomedical practitioners continued to flourish with their own funds and leaders. Needless to say, a key element for integration is strong project or national support.

A corollary to this model is that biomedical practitioners need to know about ethnomedicine so they can utilize complementary treatments. An analysis of herbal infusions given to treat diarrhea indicates that some are fairly complete rehydration solutions, requiring only an additional ingredient or two. An integrated program employing this model would provide clinics with both types of medical practices.

The syncretic model has metaphorically been described as a "belt and suspender" approach to integration. Following this approach, bio- and ethnomedical practitioners combine healing techniques, sharing each other's professional knowledge. Such was the case in the 1950s when some Kallawaya herbalists used plants and synthetic drugs that had just become popular in Bolivia, but by the 1970s, some had abandoned the synthetic drugs. For example, a world famous Kallawaya herbalist, Florentine Alvarez, was a drug salesman in the 1950s for Vita, a pharmaceutical firm in La Paz, until he realized the dangers and abuses of antibiotics and later returned to strictly natural curing (Bastien 1987:27–29). Other herbalists, however, are continuing to use synthetic drugs. Likewise, some doctors and nurses are beginning to use herbal medicines in their therapy, adding medicinal plants to their usual inventory of synthetic drugs.

The syncretic approach works best when items from either biomedicine or ethnomedicine fit into the other's etiological framework without disrupting its integrity. Desoto, Franklin, and Velasco, three Bolivian physicians incorporating both approaches, recognized the curative effects of certain medicinal plants and were able to substitute these remedies for expensive synthetic drugs, but they used them according to the biomedical paradigm. In contrast, Alvarez realized the curative effects of antibiotics at first, but later argued that they were hard to fit into hot and cold categories and that they were too drastic and an unnatural intervention into the healing process.

Whereas the healing context for biomedical practitioners is science and technology, the context for ethnomedical practitioners is an ethnoscience preserved by and unique to the culture. The syncretic approach often negates the fact that ethnomedical systems are based on complex epistemological, ethnophysiological, ethnobotanical, and cosmological systems. These ethnosciences are grounded in a long-term adaptation to the environment and a compilation of carefully observed experiences and collective wisdom. Kallawaya herbalists, for example, use over 1,000 medicinal plants within a healing context that interrelates the plant's known active ingredients with assumptions about how the body works and the body's interrelationship to nature and the cosmos (Bastien 1987:67–93; Girault 1984). The objectives of any health project should be to show how different medical systems can adapt to each other and how healthy characteristics of each system can be articulated into the workings of the other without reducing the one into the other.

Toward an Articulation Model of Integration

The approach to integration advocated within this book is one of articulation or a modified autonomy model. This model advocates maintaining the ethnoscience and cultural integrity of ethnomedicine and accommodating the folk knowledge of its practitioners. This approach not only respects and recognizes the value of ethnomedicine as being linked to environmentally adaptive strategies, as well as deeply rooted beliefs, but also assists its practitioners in improving their therapeutic efforts with biomedical practices that are economically and environmentally adaptive, consonant with cultural beliefs, and sensitive to their experiences of illnesses. Articulation implies a culturally sensitive understanding of the ethnomedical system and its assumptions (body concepts, cosmology, etiology, and ethnopharmacology), practices, and ecology of the region to which it is adapted. Knowledge of these structural features is essential in order to fit some technique from biomedicine into the system.

Consequently, articulation requires research into the ecological and cultural features of ethnomedicine. To counteract those doctors and nurses who underestimate the complexity of non-Western medical systems and believe them to be the result of ignorance and lack of education, anthropologists and other international health professionals have amply documented the coherence of logic and therapeutic value within these systems (Bastien 1987; Finkler 1985; Kleinman 1980; Rubel et al. 1984; WHO 1977; WHO and UNICEF 1978). Research is now needed on how to introduce change items into the structural framework of ethnomedical systems without making them dependent on the structure of biomedicine. We need to know: what are the underlying cognitive patterns of ethnomedical practitioners; what is the history and development of these practices; what are the political factors involved in these practices; and how do these practices interrelate to the environment and ecology? Answering these questions must be followed by the even more difficult task of assessing how proposed changes affect cultural, social, political, economic, and ecological factors within the community. Sometimes changes in health care create other problems: prenatal care has increased the population in many parts of the world and created distribution problems in many areas.

Articulation, however, works both ways, and many features of ethnomedicine must be introduced into biomedicine. By including folk healers in a health delivery system, doctors and nurses can improve their skills by comparing how healers care for the needs of the sick. Another obvious contribution of ethnomedicine to biomedicine is in the use of medicinal plants. Folk healers provide natural curing methods that are alternatives to the use of many drugs that have negative side effects. Many of these folk remedies have been tried and tested by time and people (Duke 1975:83–100).

Although most scientists recognize this, there is seldom a return of biomedical information about these plants to herbalists. Ethnobotanical research has been given little funding because scientists claim that they can synthesize cures faster than they can find them in plants. This argument, however, doesn't justify the wait of indigenous populations whose herbalists have already found cures to many diseases. Herbalists and pharmacologists can articulate the best of ethnoscience and bioscience by exchanging information on plants: herbalists can provide reputed therapeutic effects of plants through firsthand observation, and pharmacologists can test these plants for active ingredients and toxic effects.

An even stronger argument for the modified autonomous model is that many species of medicinal plants are rapidly disappearing with the destruction of tropical forests, that herbalists have knowledge of these plants, that ethnoscience is important to the preservation of this region, and that these plants are potential cures for peoples of temperate climates. In South China, for example, 6,500 medicinal plants are vanishing because of people's preference for pills. Reporting on plants with reputed therapeutic effects by herbalists and the testing of these plants for active ingredients and toxicity by biomedical technicians is an example of articulation that respects autonomy and utilizes each other's science and methodology. Moreover, it is recognizing the libraries of medicine found in the ethnosciences of herbalists throughout the world.

Government Policy

Articulation of biomedicine and ethnomedicine needs the support of national agencies and governments that have policies for incorporating indigenous practitioners. The United States Agency for International Development (USAID) has adopted the following guidelines pertaining to the training and utilization of ethnomedical practitioners (Pillsbury 1979:26). First, doctors, nurses, and health administrators should recognize that folk healers are already a major community-based health-care resource for rural and low-income urban populations and that, in many communities, folk healers are the only providers of health care. Even where doctors and nurses are present, they are often bypassed in favor of ethnomedical practitioners because doctors and nurses prove ineffective due to their misunderstandings and oppositions to ethnomedicine and its practitioners. Second, health workers should encourage and support developing-country initiatives and efforts in training and utilizing ethnic healers for primary health care. Third, health planners should urge greater understanding of and attention to ethnomedicine and other locally prevailing sociocultural practices in the training of all categories of health workers and in the planning and implementation of all health-care projects and programs. USAID/ Bolivia has followed these guidelines and been successful in using folk healers for several of its funded health projects (Proyecto Britanico–Cardenal Maurer in the Department of Chuquisaca, Project Concern in the Departments of Oruro and Cochabamba, and Save the Children in the Department of La Paz).

Even though directors of USAID in Bolivia try to incorporate ethnomedicine into primary health care, administrators and doctors at lower levels of administration resist articulation. In Bolivia and elsewhere, doctors reject ethnomedical practitioners and will exclude them from primary health care unless they receive strong mandates from funding agencies and ministries of health.

One way that national governments have helped the process of articulation is by establishing research institutes. At least twenty-one countries, universities, and governments have established institutes of ethnomedicine for research and treatment. These include Burma, China, Ethiopia, Ghana, India, Mali, Nepal, Nigeria, Senegal, the Commonwealth of Independent States, and Zaire (WHO 1977). The World Health Organization is involved in establishing a number of collaborating centers in the different disciplines that constitute ethnomedicine, and, at present, twenty-one have been designated: five in Africa, three in the Americas, two in Europe, one in the eastern Mediterranean, eight in the western Pacific, and two in Southeast Asia (Akerele 1987:180).

Research in ethnomedicines not only contributes to the health care of rural populations but may also serve the national economy. A World Health Organization team visiting a sub-Saharan and western African country found that 40 percent of the country's drug budget was needed to import three drugs (30 percent was spent for ampicillin alone) (Catsambas and Foster 1986:31). However, scientists at the University of Dakar, Senegal, have produced and tested a cough syrup derived from the native gueira plant, which is reported to be just as effective as codeine-based drugs imported from Europe and North America. This cough syrup saves Senegal an estimated $421,000 a year in foreign exchange. Another promising discovery at Dakar is a low-cost laxative derived from the local yam plant, which could decrease the annual drug-import bill by another $210,000 (Land 1986:3).

Realizing the significant subjective and objective roles of ethnomedical healers and the medical and economic benefit from research in indigenous medicine is an accomplishment, but it is not enough. There is a need to design national primary health-care programs that successfully involve ethnomedical practitioners. We need to know how members of the formal health services can work with ethnomedical practitioners for the benefit of the population; how native healers can be given responsibility and leadership roles in national health services; how health professionals can be sensitized and trained so that they support the national ethnomedical program; how health legislation concerning ethnomedicine should be reviewed; how countries can develop national drug policies that include herbal remedies; how up-to-date research and development policies in ethnomedicine can be formulated; and how ethnomedical research can be financed and encouraged.

Due to the complex nature of cultural adaptation and innovation and the enormous variation in local and regional ethnomedical systems, there is no single or simple approach to the problem of how to involve ethnomedical practitioners in national health systems, especially at the primary health-care level. Dedicated and sincere action on the part of all concerned is required to foster a collective effort to generate and implement policies best suited to any country. As Libbet Crandon-Malamud (1987) has observed: rather than dying out, indigenous medical systems are adapting to change, and medical pluralism, rather than pure biomedicine, will replace earlier medical resource use.

PART II
Herbalists and Shamans

OPPOSITION AND ADAPTATION TO BIOMEDICINE

3

Adaptive Strategies of Bolivian Herbalists to Biomedicine

The process of integrating ethnomedicine and biomedicine involves opposition and adaptation by their practitioners. This process is best illustrated by examining the ethnomedical practices of three Kallawaya herbalists in Bolivia and their relationships with doctors. Florentino Alvarez utilizes both ethnomedicine and biomedicine; Mario Salcedo has sanitized herbal practices to make them more biomedicinal; and Nestor Llaves has modified ethnomedicine to treat a clientele dissatisfied with biomedicine. Essential to the practice of ethnomedicine is that it be flexible, adapting to changing political, economic, social, and cultural conditions, more so than in biomedicine with its costly technology, political affiliations, and structured practice through licensing procedures and conventional medical schools (Foucault 1975). Kallawaya herbalists exhibit this required flexibility by their adaptation to the geographical, social, political, and economic environment of Bolivia.

The Kallawaya ethnic group has about 128 herbalists who employ more than a thousand medicinal plants, 25 to 30 percent of which provide effective cures (Girault 1984:22; 1987). Effective here means according to measurements using biomedical methodology. Another 30 percent are likely "effective" using another yardstick and may be important in healing. These herbalists are renowned throughout Argentina, Bolivia, Peru, and Chile as very skilled healers. They employ elaborate rituals in their healing (see Bastien 1978; Girault 1988; Oblitas Poblete 1978; and Rosing 1990).

Although Kallawayas speak Quechua, Spanish, and some Aymara, the herbalists use a secret language for curing, *machaj-juyai,* which means language of colleagues (Girault 1989; Oblitas Poblete 1968). Although this language is rapidly disappearing, it had an estimated 12,000 words. Herbalists speak it principally to exclud[e] in curing rituals. *Machaj-juyai* is a hybrid language [with a] lexicon mostly of Puquina words and a Quechua g[rammar] 1972). As Puquina disappeared in the seventeenth cent[ury] continued to use Puquina words with a Quechua gr[ammar] about plants and medicinal paraphernalia.

47

In 1969 I began research among the Kallawaya and have continued until the present (Bastien 1973, 1978, 1982, 1983, 1985, 1987; Bastien et al. 1990).

The Kallawaya live in Province Bautista Saavedra, Department of La Paz, Bolivia, which borders on Peru, northwest of Lake Titicaca. Charazani is the provincial capital. Approximately thirteen thousand Kallawayas live in Bautista Saavedra (975 square miles), an area the size of the state of Delaware. Population density is 13.3 people per square mile. Although many Kallawayas have moved to cities, the population has not decreased much due to improved health and birth rates. Bautista Saavedra is located north of the Cordillera Real (Oriental) in the foothills of the Apolobamba mountains, also called the Carabaya mountains. Water from Lake Titicaca and glaciers in the Apolobamba mountains feed Río Charazani and Río Calaya, which flow east to join the Mapiri and Beni rivers of the Amazon. The Charazani and Calaya rivers form a system of high and medium valleys where the Kallawaya live at elevations between 2,700 and 5,000 m, above the rain forests of the Yungas area and below the regions of permafrost. Their proximity to high mountain and tropical ecological zones provides access to many plants, animals, and minerals used in their curing procedures.

These rivers and valleys create natural boundaries for an *ayllu,* an ecological, cultural, and social unit of Kallawaya society. Tributaries flowing into the Charazani and Calaya rivers and form triangulated land masses with various ecological levels. The Kallawaya, and many other Andeans as well, distinguish their communities according to the mountain on which the community is located. The mountains are the *ayllus* and each one has three major levels: low, central, and high, where basically corn (cereals), potatoes, and llamas are produced. After the Bolivian Agrarian Reform (1954), the *ayllu* system was diminished, with prominence given to separate communities and Bolivian political units (cantons, provinces, and peasant syndicates). The Kallawaya have nine *ayllus:* Amarete, Chajaya, Chari, Chullina, Curva, Inca, Calaya, Kaata, and Upinhuaya.

The Kallawaya are horticulturalists and herders. A family lives in three small adobe buildings (5 m by 4 m), one for cooking, one for sleeping, and one for storage. The buildings form three sides of a courtyard, which is enclosed by a wall with a gate and is where family members weave, raise chickens and guinea pigs, and congregate. Burros, pigs, and sheep are kept in open corrals behind the sleeping quarters. Within each *ayllu,* people in the lower communities grow maize, wheat, barley, peas, and beans on the lower slopes (3,200 to

3,500 m); those in central communities cultivate *oca* (*Oxalis crassicaulis*) and potatoes on rotated fields of the central slopes (3,500 to 4,300 m); and those of highland communities herd alpacas, llamas, and sheep on the highlands (4,300 to 5,000 m). Traditionally, *ayllu* members from the three levels exchange produce and provide each other with the necessary carbohydrates, minerals, and proteins to maintain a balanced subsistence.

Herbalists live in *ayllus* Chajaya (28); Chari (15); Curva (37), which also includes Lagunilla (13); and Inca (15). There are also herbalists in Charazani (8) and Huata Huata (12). These *ayllus* and communities have specialized in herbal medicine and are complementary to *ayllus* that have other specialties. Amarete and Upinhuaya provide potters and tool- and hatmakers for the province. According to a division of labor, the communities on each mountain specialize in some profession. The *ayllus* exchange services and supply each other as well as other parts of the central Andes with necessary resources.

For Kaatans, their *ayllu* also has metaphorical meanings: they believe their mountain has three resource areas and communities that are analogous to the human body. In brief, Kaatans relate Apacheta, Kaata, and Niñokorin—the high, central, and low communities—to the head, trunk, and legs of a human body.

The mountain-body metaphor is the unifying and holistic principle for *ayllu* Kaata. Judy, my wife, and I participated as members of the Marcelino Yanahuaya family in twelve rituals that dealt with sickness, death, lineage, and land (Bastien 1973). In some way, every ritual centered around the mountain metaphor. Sickness, for example, is cured by symbolically putting the body of the mountain together. Marriage rituals gather together people and produce from three levels of the mountain to symbolize that marriage unites the people of the mountain. Metaphorically, then, agriculture, health, and social principles correspond to a mountain seen as a human body with its three parts (Bastien 1978:xix).

An *ayllu* and its relationships are bases for cognitive and cultural understandings of how Kallawayas perceive their bodies and how they deal with sicknesses. Most important, ethnomedical practitioners perform rituals that are enacted, shared, and negotiated discourses concerned with the integration (health) or disintegration (sickness) of bodies, communities, resources, and mountains (see Bastien 1978:129–70; 1987:67–76). An ethnological comprehension of this system provides a basis for not only understanding Kallawaya ethnomedicine per se but also seeing how it functions within an ecological and cultural context. This contextual knowledge is necessary for incorporating ethnomedicine with biomedicine in Bolivia and in other countries as well.

The Traveling Herbalists

Kallawaya herbalists, many of whom now live in cities, serve community members by bringing them medicines and produce from other places. Reliance on the exchange of goods between urban herbalists and rural peasants is important as a buffer in a region of unpredictable weather and frequent crop failure. Only one-quarter of the adult male population in Chajaya and Curva are herbalists; other individuals provide them with a support system: gathering herbs, repairing roads, providing food, and maintaining their animals, land, and households. Women take care of the animals and farm while men are absent on herbal trips, usually during the nonproductive part of the agricultural year. Children herd sheep and work in the fields soon after they begin to walk.

For centuries, Kallawayas traded medicinal knowledge among themselves and other Andean groups. Various villages had assigned trade routes for their herbalists: those from Curva traveled to Cochabamba, Oruro, Potosí, and Sucre in Bolivia; Arequipa, Peru; and northern Argentina. Those from Chajaya and Kanlaya traveled through the Central Highlands of Peru to Lima and up the coast to Ecuador, at times reaching the Panama Canal. *Ayllu* Calaya harvested coca in the Yungas and marketed it in the densely populated areas of the Puna. This international trade has decreased because of difficulties crossing borders, settlement in urban centers, and changing markets.

The Long History of Herbalists

Kallawaya herbalists follow a long history of healing and are part of an Andean ethnomedical system (Bastien 1985). Kallawayas were purveyors of medicines during the Tiahuanaco cultures (A.D. 400–1145), Mollo culture (1145–1438), Inca Empire (1438–1532), Spanish Conquest (1532–1825), and the Bolivian Republic (1825–present). As early as the Tiahuanaco period, Kallawayas practiced trephination, reshaped craniums, and used enemas, snuff trays, and medicinal plants from lowland regions (Wassén 1972). Throughout Mollo culture, Kallawayas built elaborate cisterns as burials for their ancestors who were prominent in ritual and herbal powers (Arellano López 1978). During the Inca Empire, they carried the chair of the Inca (Guaman

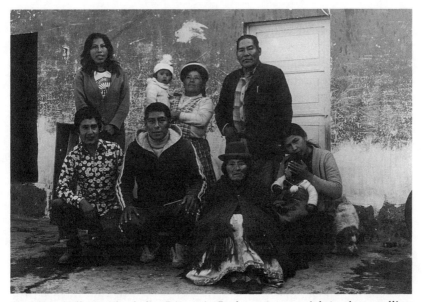

Traveling Kallawaya herbalist Dionecio Pacheco (upper right), whose calling takes him to Argentina. His wife, also an herbalist, treats patients in La Paz while he is away.

Poma de Ayala 1936:331), traveled up and down the Andes, and learned the pharmacopoeias of many Andean groups. After the Spanish conquest, Kallawayas lost large parts of their land and were moved to villages. Covertly, they continued worshipping their ancestors and earth shrines, but they also learned about European medicinal plants (Saignes 1984). After independence in 1825, the Republican period ushered in the rise of the mestizos in Charazani, who considered themselves a class apart from the peasants of the surrounding *ayllus*. Some of these mestizos became herbalists and competed with peasant herbalists. To avoid their influence and competition, Kallawayas from communities of Curva and Chajaya traveled long distances throughout Argentina, Chile, Ecuador, and Peru. The herbalists of each *ayllu* had distinct trade routes that they protected by mutual agreement among the elders. Through this widespread travel, they had become world famous by the turn of the twentieth century.

During the first half of the twentieth century, there were few doctors and clinics in rural Bolivia. Native practitioners healed the sick and there was little competition between them and doctors. Synthetic drugs were unavailable to peasants, who used medicinal plants. In 1904, for instance, Paloma, an herbalist from Achacachi, performed trephination on Francisca Calderon, who had had her skull fractured in a fight (Bandelier 1904). With a pocketknife, Paloma cut an oblong hole in the temporal ridge, released the fluid, and sewed the skin over the wound. Learning of this successful surgery with rudimentary instruments, doctors from La Paz presented Paloma with a surgical kit that he never used, preferring his pocketknife. This is an *early* example of attempts to collaborate between practitioners of ethnomedicine and biomedicine. Even though Paloma practiced with outdated techniques, he and other herbalists, such as the Kallawaya, were the only medical practitioners available to Andean peasants at the time.

During the nineteenth and early twentieth centuries, the Kallawaya acquired notoriety for certain cures. For example, Fawcett relates how Carlos Franck's daughter was cured by a Kallawaya, Pablo Alvarez (Oblitas Poblete 1969:19). She was crippled, and German doctors in Lima who had performed four hip operations had failed to cure her. Alvarez was successful in a week with a treatment of compresses and medicinal plants. Cures such as this one fostered the reputation of the Kallawaya to such a degree that they were sent to the Panama Canal to cure workers of yellow fever, which they did with *quina cascarilla* (quinine bark). In 1889, Kallawaya herbalists got worldwide attention when they sent a list of their pharmacopoeia to the Eighth World Exposition of Paris. Doctor Nicanor Iturralde and Eugenio Guinault studied the list and classified the plants according to botanical species and pharmacological uses by Kallawayas. Commenting on their work, Carlos Bravo (1918:167–72) wrote that this was a profound study that included many native plants and information needed for world health. Bravo criticized the authors for not readily accepting the medicinal qualities of these plants: "If the lowly, ignorant Indians are cured by these plants, what more evidence do we need?"

Kallawaya acclaim became so widespread during this period that people came from other countries of South America and Europe to be treated for diseases that had been diagnosed as incurable. Kallawaya herbal medicine assumed legendary dimensions, partially because of the herbalists' mysterious practices, transient activities, and knowledge of medicinal plants. Moreover, herbalists employed magic, ritual, and prayers in their healing sessions, which gave them an aura of shamanism. These factors made it difficult to validate the authenticity of reputed cures. Incurables thought of them as their healing saviors. Realistically, however, the Kallawaya refused to treat patients who were likely to die or could not be cured by their methods. Consequently, their success rate was higher than that of doctors who accepted patients on their deathbeds. The herbalists' trademark was, and still is, an elaborately woven shoulder bag for herbs neatly wrapped in cloths to distinguish them. Kallawaya herbalists were called *Qolla Kapachayuh* (Lords of the Medicine Bag) and their *ayllus* were called *Qollahuaya* (Place of Herbs). (Kallawaya is an alternative spelling for Qollahuaya.)

Suppression of Lords of the Medicine Bag

Toward the second half of the twentieth century, doctors and pharmacists campaigned against the "backward" practices of herbalists, depicting them as obstacles to scientific medicine. Doctors, nurses, and auxiliary nurses started serving peasants after the Bolivian Agrarian Reform in 1954. Herbalists were prohibited from practicing medicine in many places. Some were arrested, tried, and imprisoned for short sentences. Others were classified as *brujos*, witches. In order to avoid these criticisms, some herbalists, such as Mario Salcedo of La Paz, used only empirical cures and discontinued prayers, symbols, and rituals in healing sessions. Others practiced covertly. This persecution brought a decline in the number of herbalists, because as one old herbalist told me, "Why should I educate my son to be an herbalist, a profession of Gypsies."

Another factor for the decline of herbalism during the 1940s and 1950s was the advent of synthetic medicines, the "miracle drugs." Antibiotics such as penicillin and streptomycin cured syphilis and tuberculosis, both common in Bolivia, much faster than did *cola de caballo* (shavegrass) and *salvia grande* (sage). The emerging classes of Westernized Bolivians believed that modern medicine had replaced their remedies from the countryside. Pharmaceutical companies, which previously had relied on herbs and herbalists for their prescriptions, now imported synthetic drugs at greater costs and much greater profits. They became competitors with herbalists, who lacked the advantages of packaging, public endorsement, and advertisement. In fact, pharmaceutical companies, such as Vita and Inti, in Bolivia had developed about forty pharmaceutical products from herbal recipes of Kallawaya herbalists, providing no patent rights. Although this appears to have legitimized the use of herbs, pharmaceutical products from herbs were given new names, references to plant sources were omitted, and herbal suppliers were minimally paid. Because of this exploitation, herbalists refused to collaborate with pharmaceutical companies in research. The lesson learned is that compensation is necessary for herbalists whose plants are used commercially. Patent rights need to be extended to herbalists.

An example of infringement of property rights for commercial gain happened recently. The musical group Kaoma stole a song, "Llorando se Fue," from another musical group, Los Karkas, and made millions from it. They had changed the lyrics to Portuguese and given it a lambada rhythm. Nonetheless, Los Karkas won the lawsuit as having prior rights to the song and received compensation. Relevant here is that pharmaceutical companies are violating intellectual property rights of many herbalists who continue to own rights to discoveries of herbal remedies. Unless these herbalists are compensated, lawsuits will be forthcoming.

By the middle of the twentieth century, many Kallawayas had moved to cities and abandoned their craft; those who did continue practicing medicine dressed in Western clothing, forgot their language, and accepted biomedicine. There was a sharp decline in the number of medicinal plants used in curing. Old-time herbalists used an average of 300 medicinal plants, whereas younger herbalists were by 1960 using around 80 plants. Herbalists made fewer trips and many illnesses were dealt with more effectively by synthetic drugs. When I visited herbalists from 1963 through 1985, they were cautious and reticent about disclosing their practice for fear that they would be persecuted by the Ministry of Rural Health. In 1979 Pastor Llaves, a noted Kallawaya herbalist in Cochabamba, said that he had been refused permission to visit his patients in the hospital and had also been arrested for herbal practices.

Renewal of Herbalism

During my fieldwork from 1985 until the present, Kallawaya herbalists were less reticent, and proudly talked about their practices. The waning herbal tradition began waxing in 1985 when Bolivians and others throughout the Western world began rediscovering the value of medicinal plants. Bolivians, especially peasants, could little afford synthetic drugs and feared their side effects. First-generation Aymara Indians received penicillin injections with high rates of success and few reactions, but second and subsequent generations had lower rates of success and substantial reactions.

Moreover, there was a growing hostility to Westernization and capitalization of Bolivia. Before Victor Paz ascended to the presidency in 1985, cocaine cartels had brought corruption, and either bought or opposed regimes. Tin mines were closed in Oruro by 1985,

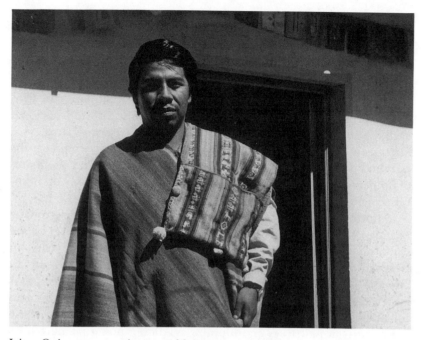

Jaime Quispe, twenty-six years old, is an aspiring Kallawaya herbalist in Valle-grande, Bolivia. A former medical student, he discontinued his studies because he felt more adept at ethnomedicine. His father is a famous herbalist. I trained Jaime in ethnobotany and anthropological field methods.

vastly increasing unemployment, and inflation had reached 29,800 percent. Effects on the poor and middle classes were great, with their salaries light years behind the rate of inflation. As soon as workers were paid, they rushed to buy merchandise before their money devalued at 80 percent a day. Merchants stopped buying and selling goods, many closing shop to move to other countries, as also did members of the professional classes.

Bolivians became disillusioned with the high cost of biomedicine and its dependence upon international economic forces. The price of imported pharmaceutical products rose with inflation: in 1984 the cost of a penicillin injection was upwards of U.S. $10, several days' wages for peasants. Doctors and nurses were frequently on strike. These economic factors forced Bolivians to develop appropriate technologies from internal natural resources. Bolivians began look-ing more to their own traditions for solutions and less to products from the industrialized countries. Bolivians resorted to herbs, herb-alists, and other ethnomedical practitioners.

Herbal medicines increased in demand, as did herbalists and

herbal vendors. Although the population of La Paz tripled between 1965 and 1985, the number of herbal stalls in La Paz increased from 30 to 130. The herbal market in Oruro is one of the largest business endeavors in the Department of Oruro, estimated as a multimillion dollar operation (Greg Rake, pers. com. 1986). One female herbal vendor travels to China to trade Bolivian medicinal plants for Chinese herbs (Oscar Velasco, pers. com. 1986). An international exchange of folk remedies brings medicinal plants from Africa, Asia, Europe, and other parts of Latin America to Bolivia, which can be purchased from herbal vendors throughout the country. Estimates of 60 percent to 70 percent of the Bolivian population rely on natural remedies.

Another reason for the increase in herbalism is the growing resentment of Bolivians toward doctors who perform surgery, are sometimes unsuccessful, and charge excessive fees. For years, in Bolivia the two routes to gentlemanliness and legitimacy were medicine and law. Now, doctors in Bolivia no longer have this prestigious and wealthy role compared to doctors in the United States and Europe—one reason why many doctors have emigrated to these countries—nor do they monopolize medicine now that herbalists are popular.

Certain problems arose with the rising popularity of herbal curing. Improperly trained herbalists tried to cash in on the booming trade. Claiming to be Kallawayas, these impostors cheated the sick with concoctions of narcotic and toxic plants. The Kallawaya Mario Salcedo observed that peasants come to La Paz to be treated by doctors who are unable to cure them, so they resort to poorly trained city herbalists who deceive them with plants and magic. They finally return to their villages to be treated by country herbalists.

Unemployment also contributed to the increase in the number of herbalists. Out of work, some adopted the herbal profession which, unfortunately, because of its esoteric nature, could easily be manipulated to "con" already desperate and vulnerable patients. Furthermore, the number of herbal books increased, and courses in traditional medicine were offered by members of the Escuela Nacional de Salud Pública and the Sociedad Boliviana de Medicina Natural (SBMN). Mario Salcedo lectured on uses of plants (see Bastien 1987:10–11, 29–32). Walter Alvarez, M.D., son of a Kallawaya herbalist, discussed pathology and herbal cures. And Jaime Zalles, a homeopathologist, and Jaime Mondaca, a medical student, trained participants in certain aspects of biomedicine. These courses lasted four days, two hours each evening, and were attended by around fifteen people. Participants were charged five bolivianos (U.S. $1 = B. $2.05 = day's meals). Inappropriately, some participants considered themselves herbalists after attending one course.

The integration between herbalists and doctors in Bolivia has also improved with the increased interest in ethnomedicine. Doctors and herbalists collaborated with Servicios Múltiples de Tecnologías Apropiadas (SEMTA) in organizing several herbal and biomedical courses, one within the Kallawaya region and two outside the region. SEMTA also helped erect two buildings in the Kallawaya region, which were to become schools for aspiring herbalists, but has since abandoned the program. Herbalists and medical doctors jointly staff clinics in La Paz, El Alto, and Oruro, and plan to staff a hospital for Kallawayas of *ayllu* Amarete. Finally, there was a national symposium on ethnomedicine and biomedicine in Oruro, Bolivia, in 1985.

Legitimacy and Licensing

Mario Salcedo and Walter Alvarez suggested, as a measure to control the quality of herbalists in Bolivia, that expert herbalists should provide aspirants longer courses with qualifying exams and licenses to practice. Although they are correct in calling for measures to discriminate against unqualified herbalists, they also advocate that herbalists be licensed by the Ministry of Health (MPSSP), which is doctor controlled. As legitimacy and status become the means to control herbalists, the diversity of practices among Kallawayas will be lost. Herbalists follow a folk tradition that is subject to change and experience: it is not codified into set formulas, such as medical books, which are compilations of empirical facts and generalizations, scientifically verifiable. Kallawaya folklore is passed along from father to son and learned by practice. The effort to formalize this folklore with herbal institutes, manuals, exams, and licenses might make herbalists more uniform in their practice, but it might also inhibit the dynamic aspects of a living tradition. Herbalists would also be less flexible. Bolivia has many ethnic groups and classes of people. For Kallawayas to be effective, they must adapt their practice to these differing cultures, politics, and economics.

Doctors object to this by replying that if degrees and licenses are not required of these practitioners, how are Bolivians to know who is qualified or not. For foreigners and strangers, this is a problem, but it is not for most Bolivians, who select ethnomedical practitioners, as well as biomedical practitioners, according to reputation. The Kallawaya slowly build up their practice by successful curing rates. They also establish social ties with patients and their families. Among Kallawayas, herbalists are ranked according to expertise, so that, if asked, they will tell you who is the most noted healer, such as when they nominated Florentino Alvarez to be in charge of the ethnomedicine display in La Paz in 1956.

As a folk system, ethnomedicine has its own criteria of expertise. In the integration of herbalists, criteria found in the community can be used for evaluating their practices. The communities of Chajaya and Curva exert a controlling influence on the quality of herbalists from these villages. Elders of Chajaya require that an aspirant herbalist serve as an apprentice before curing alone. When herbalists gather at fiestas to compare herbs and cures, they criticize the less skilled so they can protect their reputation and income. Some Kallawaya herbalists offer a guarantee in the sense that they do not charge if a patient is not cured. If, however, a patient dies, they may not charge for fear of reprisals. Where members of the community do not exert much influence over ethnomedical practitioners, associations of healers may serve a similar function of regulating their practice.

For Kallawayas, an apprenticeship used to last as long as eight years, which contemporary youths consider too long for too little reward. One solution is to combine apprenticeship with book learning to facilitate the dissemination of herbal knowledge. One disadvantage of this is that more emphasis is placed on abstract information than on observation, experience, and personal contact. No known herbal study is able to contain the experiences, insights, and knowledge of a practitioner such as Florentino Alvarez. To carry on the Kallawaya tradition, long-term apprenticeships are necessary. Another disadvantage would be the structure imposed to disseminate such knowledge should the state want to control it by licensure (Libbet Crandon-Malamud, pers. com. 1990).

Syncretizeor: Florentino Alvarez

Popularity and profiteering pose problems for older Kallawaya herbalists, who fear their tradition is losing its quality. A major concern of these herbalists is that their children do not want to spend long apprenticeships learning their craft. Consider how Florentino Alvarez, a very famous Kallawaya herbalist, learned how to cure (Bastien 1987:27–29). In 1924, when Florentino was thirteen, he served as

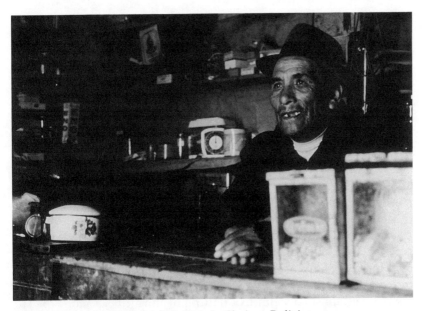

Florentino Alvarez in his herbal clinic in Chajaya, Bolivia.

an apprentice to Damian Alvarez, an accomplished herbalist who specialized in ailments of the kidneys, lungs, liver, and those related to childbirth. Damian became like a father to Florentino, teaching him the art of herbal curing. They spent months combing the countryside from their native village of Chajaya to Lima gathering plants and then visiting hamlets up and down the valleys of the Andes and across the deserts of Peru curing the sick.

When Damian died in 1926, Florentino continued his education with another famous herbalist, Manuel Redondo. Together, they traveled thousands of miles up and down the north coast of Peru and across the Andes to Kanlaya. They cured all classes of people: Indians, mestizos, Europeans. According to Florentino, Manuel cured crippled people by making them sweat with *chilca,* eucalyptus, and nettle leaves boiled in water. He cured pain in the lungs by rubbing the chest with a lotion made from animal fat, and he treated yellow fever with enemas made from quinine bark. Relatives provided Florentino and Manuel with food and lodging during the cure, which lasted from a few days to several weeks. They cured in the home and were well paid.

Florentino oscillated between ethnomedicine and biomedicine, an ambiguity that enabled him to examine and criticize both systems. At different times, he adopted nature curing with water therapy, and at others he resorted to biomedicine. Florentino frequently used elements from several alternative medicines, and was described by Doctor Harold Haley (pers. com. 1982) as being like someone who after the introduction of the belt could not abandon the security of suspenders and so wore both. This metaphor captures the insecurity of herbalists, such as Florentino, who act as bridges between traditional ethnomedicine and revolutionary biomedicine.

In 1940, Florentino temporarily abandoned the use of herbs for chemotherapeutic products from Inti and Vita. As their representative he traveled the southern route from La Paz to Santa Cruz, Argentina. He soon observed that synthesized drugs cost more and caused more side effects than did medicinal plants.

In 1942 Florentino quit his job with the pharmaceutical companies and served as an apprentice of Professor Reyes, a natural healer. Reyes had recently come from Santiago, Chile, to set up a clinic in La Paz. He taught Florentino the uses of water in healing: baths, saunas, and massages. That same year, Florentino returned to Chajaya, where he established a clinic of natural healing (clínica naturista). He constructed an adobe Turkish bath and built cabinets for medicinal plants. He also operated a small store with basic supplies of rice, sugar, soft drinks, kerosene, and candles. When he was not farming, he would sit behind a blue wooden counter and sell his supplies or discuss cures with people.

Florentino continued to travel several times a year until 1960, when he fell from a cliff and broke his foot. After this, people traveled from Argentina, Chile, Peru, and other parts of Bolivia to Chajaya to be healed by him. They made long and difficult journeys: the trip from La Paz to Chajaya is ten hours riding in the back of a large truck loaded with supplies and people. Nonetheless, ten to fifteen people visited Florentino annually to be cured. They believed that he was able to heal the incurables.

Unlike some other herbalists, Florentino was not presumptuous about his skills; he was deeply humble and admitted many failures in curing. There was no magic involved. Essentially, he was a very compassionate healer, who, if he was unable to cure someone, at least helped the person deal with his or her sickness. He also told the truth to sick people, careful not to mislead them about his abilities. This is contrary to some herbalists who claim to cure any disease, only to deceive the clientele temporarily. Florentino's humility and desire to heal diseases motivated him to continually search for cures.

As a result, Florentino enhanced the general reputation of all Kallawaya herbalists. In 1956, Victor Paz Estenssoro, president of

Bolivia, commissioned him to prepare a display of Kallawaya medicines for the Museo Casa Murillo in La Paz. Victor Paz wrote him a letter of commendation for his contributions to Andean medicine. This beautiful collection, titled *Botica Antigua*, is one tribute to Florentino and other Kallawayas. Florentino practiced in his clinic until 1981, when he died of a cerebral hemorrhage. He was survived by one adopted son, Vicente, who now farms Florentino's land. He is not an herbalist.

Florentino, the last of the great Kallawaya herbalists, stood on the threshold of the merging of ethnomedicine and biomedicine: his unique role was to be between ethnomedicine and the advance of biomedicine. He continually tried to incorporate the use of synthesized drugs with that of medicinal plants and to convince herbalists to use antibiotics (penicillin and streptomycin) for curing syphilis and tuberculosis. Once when I was suffering from a urinary infection, Florentino suspected syphilis and suggested that I have a blood test in La Paz. He also warned me, "Drugs are expensive. They calm the symptoms, but have many side effects." Florentino gathered sacks of rue (*Ruta chalapensis*) in the Chajaya region to sell to the Vita and Inti companies in La Paz, which used it for lotions to treat rheumatism (Bastien 1978:148–49). He complained that they paid him the same price as for a sack of corn—a minimal payment.

I was with Florentino in his store in Chajaya in 1980 when a commission of government officials and doctors visited him to announce that they wanted to start an herbal college and name him instructor. They complained that the villagers were not present to receive them. Florentino told them that the people were working in the fields and had no time to attend to formalities. He wanted to show them the new hospital in Charazani, but they refused to visit it and said they were primarily interested in herbal medicines of the Kallawaya. Walter Alvarez, M.D., who led the commission, was remotely related to Florentino, who considered him politically ambitious. Instead of learning herbal medicine, Walter had studied biomedicine in Cuba. Upon his return to Bolivia, he led a movement to incorporate Kallawaya ethnomedicine with biomedicine, somewhat for ethnic reasons but also to market herbal remedies once they became legitimate. After the commission left, Florentino was little impressed and astutely commented, *"palabras no más"* ("only words"). Although Florentino never explicitly expressed it, he communicated to me that to heal the sick he would share his knowledge with doctors, pharmacists, and anthropologists, but that they would benefit the most and provide him with very little in return.

Recalling how Florentino had received little in return for his knowledge, I gave him my binoculars, which he used to see the jagged, snow-crested peaks of Aqhamani, his earth shrine. He had suffered a stroke. I was somewhat able to help him by massaging his muscles, but he remained partially crippled. With the binoculars, his eyes could travel the distances he once had walked as an herbalist. Bolivian peasants have seldom gained from the exploitation of their country for medicines and drugs, such as quinine and cocaine. In return for information provided me, I have published an herbal manual in Spanish that is being used by promoters in the Department of Oruro (Bastien 1983a).

In 1984, Kallawaya herbalists acknowledged the contributions of Florentino Alvarez by dedicating an herbal book to him (SEMTA 1984). In an attempt to continue Kallawaya herbal tradition, Walter Alvarez started herbal colleges in *ayllus* Chajaya and Curva, but by 1989 these colleges were discontinued for lack of funds. Many herbalists continue the tradition, but there is a decreasing number of youths who are willing to spend years of apprenticeships learning by practice and oral traditions. There is a need for herbal colleges, books, and courses to replace some of the oral tradition that is being discontinued. Walter Alvarez was instrumental in helping the Kallawaya of *ayllu* Amarete get an integrated clinic with an herbalist and a doctor, supported by the Ministry of Health, which they had petitioned.

Florentino represents the ethnomedical practitioner that is first rejected, then exploited, and finally exonerated with honor. Walter represents the biomedical practitioner and descendant of herbalists that first rejects his tradition but then embraces it. Kallawaya herbalists, as well as scores of other ethnomedical practitioners, experience similar rejections and acceptances, depending on popularity, politics, economics, and nationalism.

Popular acceptance of ethnomedicine increases when there is a growing ethnic identity coupled with a lessening involvement with public institutions, especially those with international interests. Ethnomedical practitioners realize this and are suspicious of administrators' and politicians' motives. They are suspicious of attempts to integrate them into the biomedical system, not because they are unscientific but because they recognize exploitative relationships. Herbalists know that past endeavors to integrate them have either failed or resulted in further exploitation. The lesson learned is that for integration ethnomedical practitioners need surety of their rights and resources. Their practices need to be protected and not referred off to doctors, and patents should be given to them for new medicines.

Throughout the developing world, many doctors and nurses are similar to Walter in that running through their blood are ethno-medical traditions which they have been taught to reject and suppress. These doctors and nurses need to repair the damages they have done to themselves and to ethnomedical practitioners: disparagement of reputations, taking away of clients, and relegation to inferior roles. Herbalists like Florentino may be humble, but they are also sensitive and very proud. They resent being looked down on by a new breed of "technocrats." Biomedical knowledge, which brings power to doctors and nurses, oppresses herbalists when wrongly used. Aware of this, Kallawayas used a secret language for centuries to guard their precious herbal knowledge, but now that they are willing to share this knowledge with doctors, they want status, recognition, and recompense in return.

Sanitizer: Mario Salcedo

Another way that Kallawaya herbalists have adapted to biomedicine is by trying to act like doctors and nurses, as illustrated by Mario Salcedo. Mario is a Kallawaya herbalist who moved to La Paz, became a mestizo, and established a "respectable" clinic for middle- and upper-class Bolivians. Whereas Florentino represents a "belt and suspenders" type of integration, Mario represents a Kallawaya who tries to "sanitize" or legitimize ethnomedicine to make it scientific so it fits into biomedicine. Although he achieved respectability and legitimacy, he remained peripheral to the herbalists of Chajaya, who rejected his advice and never named him sponsor (preste) for the fiesta, and to doctors, who never permitted him to practice in the hospitals of La Paz. Like Florentino, Mario was an orphan and liminal figure; the former was firmly rooted as a peasant making overtures to biomedicine, and the latter became a mestizo emulating middle-class doctors. Bolivians classify people as mestizos when they have become Westernized or Europeanized by speaking Spanish fluently, wearing suits or dresses, being educated (or at least giving airs as such), and considering themselves superior to campesinos (peasants) and cholos (urbanized peasants). As herbalists attempt to integrate with doctors, they encounter questions of identity, as well as those of ethnicity, class, and domination.

Literacy has reduced the reliance that ethnomedical practitioners have had on oral traditions passed along as inheritance through

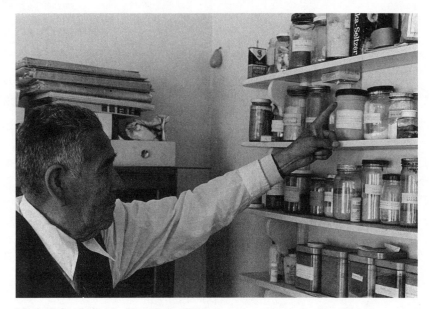

Mario Salcedo in his clinic in La Paz.

the lineage. As a result, ethnomedical practitioners can learn from books, exhibit individuality in practice, and be less dependent upon or free of controls by relatives. Mario was basically a self-taught herbalist. Born in 1908, Mario accompanied Domingo Flores on two trips, each four months long. This apprenticeship was short, so Mario began to study on his own. He learned to read and write and expanded his knowledge of curing by reading herbal books that contained popular herbal remedies from Europe and South America. At this time, vegetal drugs were the common form of treatment, so these manuals were important to Bolivian medicine. Throughout the 1930s and 1940s, Mario traveled alone and remained apart from other Kallawaya herbalists because of his knowledge and sophistication. He built up a clientele in La Paz and later remained in his La Paz clinic except when he traveled to the Kallawaya region to gather plants.

Adapting to the status of an early twentieth-century doctor, Mario exhibited self-confidence and a dogmatic view of curing. He tried to simulate the role of the medical doctor—wearing a white smock and being authoritarian, which might have given him legitimacy but which also separated him from his clients and colleagues. He attempted to legitimize his practice scientifically by debating doctors and writing articles in the newspapers. He has been instrumental in establishing cooperative clinics between doctors and herbalists in La Paz and El Alto. He avoided and openly criticized Kallawayas for curing with magic and ritual because he advocated an ethnoscience of Kallawaya healing. Kallawayas in Chajaya resented his superior attitude and ignored his criticism, which they associated with the oppressive class of mestizos in Charazani. Moreover, peasants who were tenants on his land in Chajaya harvested plants for him at low wages.

Doctors respected Mario as an old-time herbalist with professional expertise, different from other Kallawayas, especially the itinerant ones of Calle Sagarnaga in La Paz. Doctors mentioned Mario as an example of how herbalists could be integrated into health programs by a redefinition of the herbalist's role to become more technical, professional, and scientific. However, this modification increased the impersonality and aloofness between him and his patients. Although this change communicates professional skills to clients, it also gives them a sense of powerlessness and lessens their participation in the therapeutic process. Moreover, Mario might have thrown out the baby with the bath water when he discarded the magical and ritual paraphernalia of herbal curing that may have had more indirect curative effects than the active ingredients of plants.

Donald Joralemon (1986) points out in his study of Peruvian *curanderos'* curing rituals in two distinct communities that the contrast between active engagement and passive participation is attributed to the social context of the ritual location from which patients are drawn. Patients as well as specialists contribute to the modification of folk-healing practices in changed social and cultural circumstances. But, in regard to Mario's case, patients have not transformed his transactions with them as much as have his efforts to appear "professional." Herbalists I interviewed had a lower image of their profession than did doctors, with the exception of Mario, who thought he was better than most doctors and had to prove it by acting like a doctor.

Pressures for herbalists to be more "scientific" and to act like doctors may work to bring them closer to the dominant medical establishment, but it also may limit what they have to offer to total health care. A vital contribution of herbalists to biomedicine is personalized therapy and communication with their patients, involving them in the healing process if only by manipulating symbols and performing rituals. Elsewhere I have shown that there are two interrelated systems at work within Kallawaya ethnomedicine: the empirical effects of medicinal plants and how these physical factors fit into body concepts, which I have described as a topographical-hydraulic ethnophysiology (Bastien 1985). Herbalists most effectively can cure within the cultural context of how plants are understood and related to their ethnophysiology. An analogy would be if a biomedical practitioner with an office lined with diplomas, expensive equipment, and technicians diagnosed a patient by using coca leaves and prescribed some herbs. Conversely, when herbalists act like doctors, patients are confused because they have other expectations for herbalists. There is a surplus of doctors in La Paz and many are more reasonable than Mario Salcedo.

When herbalists and doctors diagnose and treat the same illness, there is frequently a problem because they do not agree as to the cause or nature of the illness, and even less to the treatment. Illnesses take on social, cultural, psychological, as well as biological meanings, which are discussed between practitioners and patients. Mario checks the urine and pulse and questions the patient about behavior and diet, which he considers important causes of illnesses. A close follower of hot/cold etiology, Mario attributes the causes of diseases to imbalances of diet and temperature. For example, he diagnosed a case of Bell's palsy, with which I had been sick years before, to have been caused by eating cold cuts of pork and lying on damp ground after playing tennis. Even though this had happened in 1959 and I had been treated by doctors and physical therapists, Mario claimed that he could cure my residual paralysis with herbs, diet, and physical therapy. Unfortunately, I did not have time to pursue the cure. Ethnomedical practitioners advertise cures for illnesses, which biomedical practitioners cannot because the former assume different causes of sickness and health from the latter. Differences in diagnosis and treatment between ethno- and biomedicine need to be understood and respected by doctors and herbalists for an integrated health program. This approach enhances both practices by including more aspects in the therapeutic process.

Granted that some of the Kallawaya practice is "scientifically sound" and founded on material and efficient causality, a large part is not, such as divinations for discussing social conflicts, rituals for relieving mental illnesses, and amulets for recovering losses. These techniques affect psychological and social factors that are important for healing. An important conclusion is that in order to collaborate with doctors, herbalists should not be pressured to use only medicinal plants, to defend the validity of their cures, and to abandon ritual cures.

Traditionalist: Nestor Llaves

Another way that ethnomedical practitioners have adapted to biomedicine is by filling in aspects of health care that biomedical practitioners do not include. As in many parts of the world, Bolivians
depend upon herbal, ritual, divinatory, and group therapeutics.
Although Mario legitimized the role of Kallawaya herbalist, he discarded some therapeutic practices. Herbal curing is a complex art
that includes a combination of physiological, psychological, spiritual, and symbolic factors. Herbalists frequently cure not because of
their medicine but because of their overall influence on the patient's
well-being.

Nestor Llaves, however, has extended the role of herbalist to
include aspects of *espiritistas* and diviners. Nestor is a Kallawaya herbalist and ritualist from *ayllu* Curva who has a clinic in La Paz. By
having a small stature and protruding stomach and engaging in
magical activity, he resembles Ekeko, the dwarf divinity of good fortune in the Andes. In reality, Nestor is about as rich as Ekeko, being
the owner of a six-ton Toyota truck, a school bus, two homes, and a
large farm in Curva. More than Mario and much more than Florentino, Nestor has built a thriving business of healing the sick in La
Paz. All classes of people consult with him concerning spiritual, psychological, and physical ailments. He deals with witchcraft, theft,
depression, hatred, unrequited love, divination, burial of the dead,
séances, and diseases. Nestor has a flexible style: treating physical
symptoms with natural remedies, supernatural disharmonies with
rituals, and psychological upsets with a combination of psychoanal-
ysis and counseling. He treats forty patients a day. The success of his
practice demonstrates that people want to be treated by psychological, supernatural, and cultural techniques along with empirical
methods of curing.

Nestor was born in 1913 in Curva to Manuel Llaves and Matiasa
Pérez. His father traveled as an herbalist to Argentina, Brazil, Chile,
Ecuador, and Peru. He died from a heart attack when Nestor was
thirteen. The following year, Nestor began learning the herbal profession from his great-grandfather, Lorenzo Llaves, and his grand-
father, Andres Llaves. Nestor, as well as other Kallawaya herbalists
from Curva, traveled frequently to Argentina between 1929 and 1944.
The people from Curva traveled this trade route, whereas those
from Chajaya traveled mostly through Peru and up the coast to
Colombia. Herbalists made contacts along these routes, establishing

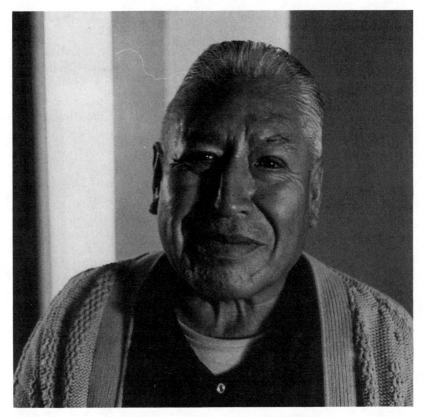

Nestor Llaves, a spiritualist as well as herbalist, has adapted traditional Kallawaya ethnomedicine to the needs of urban migrants and *cholos*.

a network of resource exchange between the various regions. This
was one way Kallawayas increased their herbal knowledge.

In 1945 Nestor stopped traveling to Argentina, and in 1946 started
a clinic in La Paz near the crowded market section of Calle Buenos
Aires after he purchased, through connections, a license from the
Municipality of the City of La Paz—but not from the Ministry of
Health as had Mario—to operate a business. Around the same time,
other Kallawaya herbalists moved to La Paz, abandoned their profession, and became jewelers, merchants, and truckers (see Bastien
1987:22–26). They established a powerful *cholo* network in La Paz connected with the Kallawaya region (see Bastien 1987:36–37 for urban/
rural ties). Also differing from Mario, who aspired to be a member of
the hispanicized mestizo class, Nestor fit into the large *cholo* class of
La Paz.

Cholos(as) are peasants who have moved to the city, still speak

Aymara or Quechua, and whose men wear pants, shirts, jackets, and occasionally a poncho to keep warm and whose women wear the traditional skirt, *pullera,* and hat (either the derby or Puritan stove). *Cholos* are a broker mercantile class who do business with *campesinos* (peasants) in the countryside and mestizos in the city. Like Nestor, *cholos* have made some interesting adaptations to the class system in La Paz: *cholo* truckers have built houses in upper-class neighborhoods that are similar in outside architecture to other houses in the area, but inside, the houses are arranged like a peasant's hut with very little furniture, stacks of supplies, and animals and children everywhere. Although not legitimately recognized as members of the mestizo class, *cholos* control a large part of the Bolivian economy, especially contraband, transportation, and trucking, and are a significant political force.

At first, Nestor's clinic was a one-room adobe hut near the crowded streets of Buenos Aires where peasants and *cholos* do business. Nestor walked the streets wearing his poncho and medicine bag, advertising himself as a Kallawaya. Slowly, people began coming to his house, sometimes only two or three a week, to consult about spiritual and physiological matters. These people told other people, and his reputation spread. By 1970, he had built a two-story apartment with reception rooms for his clients on Calle Pioneros de Rochdale.

He works ten hours a day, with all classes of people consulting him for superstitious, supernatural, psychological, and physiological reasons. He heals the warts of peasants and the headaches of generals. When the Pope was ill in 1982, some *cholos* wanted to send Nestor to Rome. He charges "Whatever you can afford," and receives whatever is appropriate because he is good at shaming cheapskates as well as generous to the poor. Rooms of his house are loaded with goods, from Swiss army knives to guinea pigs. Until recently, he drank excessively, being intoxicated for days at a time. Although this inconvenienced patients, it apparently did not discredit his practice, because they would wait until he sobered up. On several intoxicated occasions, he confided to me that he drank because he dealt with so much suffering in people's lives, continually listening to their problems. When I last visited Nestor in 1990, his wife had just died, and he had stopped drinking several years ago. He was very sad and together we prayed for his wife. He then began seeing patients; it was 7:00 A.M. and already a line had formed to visit him.

In his medical practice, Nestor combines several roles: spiritist, diviner, and herbalist. According to him, spiritists (*ch'amakani* in

Aymara) cure with prayers that intercede with the powers of the sacred places or earth shrines *(mallkus)*. Spiritists enter into a trance to negotiate an exchange with the dead so that, instead of taking the life of the sick person, the dead will be satisfied with the life of a chicken or llama. The number of talented spiritists and diviners has decreased in Bolivia, perhaps because these roles require an intuitive and mystical life-style that has become less important with modernization. The best spiritists are found in remote highland villages, where they live apart and spend long periods meditating about mountains, streams, the sun, and stars.

Because *cholos* still seek diviners to predict and deal with their earth shrines and spiritists to uncover unknown facts, ambitious Bolivians have adopted this practice with a limited amount of skill. Nestor has adopted some spiritist practices. He has a small chapel with a skull where he performs intercessions. Although he conducts wakes for the dead, he does not attempt to converse with them. He also tries to figure out the psychic causes of bad fortune, but says he lacks the psychic intuitions of a spiritist. As a diviner, Nestor diagnoses the patient by reading coca leaves and tarot cards. He does this principally to examine the possibilities and to authenticate his diagnosis. If the coca leaves, a divine plant, agree with his diagnosis, then the patient more readily accepts Nestor's opinion: there is a cultural validity to his opinion and treatment.

The intermingling of cultural symbols and clinical techniques is important for curing peasants, and Nestor is skilled at this. Nestor, however, like a diviner for agricultural rituals, uses his empirical skills to figure out what is wrong. He reads the pulse in an elaborate way, determining whether the blood is fast, slow, wet, or dry. He also examines urine and has a long list of questions concerning the person's well-being. He is a skilled counselor. For example, he employs fright to scare people out of depression and reinforcement to relax severely anxious people. He uses rosaries, holy pictures, holy water, crucifixes, incense, and amulets.

Mario Salcedo criticized Nestor and said that herbalists should dedicate themselves exclusively to the use of natural means to avoid the accusation that they are magical curers. The paradox is that Mario is a victim of cultural imperialism, yet proudly adheres to the fact that he is a Kallawaya herbalist. Whereas Nestor—also a very skilled herbalist—uses the devices of spiritists and diviners to cure his patients in a cultural context. Nestor realizes the importance of cultural context and claims that this is what the *cholos* want him to do. They ask him to pray over them, to perform rituals to feed the earth shrines, and to divine their fortune. He is smart enough to adapt to the clinical needs of the *cholo* class. Adapting to the needs of his clients, Nestor treats urban migrants: people rooted in Andean culture and befuddled by the urban industrial poverty of La Paz. *Cholos* are more concerned than mestizos in looking for links with their Andean heritage. Nestor is a mediator between the old and new ways.

In regard to class, Nestor is more realistic than Mario. Nestor admits that legitimizing his herbal trade to fit into the dominant biomedical system and mestizo class limits his practice and provides less economic gain than adapting Andean ethnomedical roles. As a result, he is wealthier than most doctors in La Paz. He treats clientele from other ethnic groups and classes. If he had tried to become a mestizo herbalist like Mario, he would have been a small fish in a big pond. Nester, however, no longer wants to be associated with the *campesino* class of Curva as did his wife, who, when dying, asked to be buried in Curva, near the land she had farmed and her earth shrine. A *Paceño* and *cholo*, Nestor purchased a funeral plan and will be buried in the cemetery wall of La Paz.

Different Strokes for Different Folks

The diverse styles of Florentino, Mario, and Nestor represent how Kallawayas have integrated their herbal practices with biomedicine. For all classes, Florentino oscillated between biomedicine and ethnomedicine, finally concentrating on natural cures and using biomedicine only when necessary. For upper- and middle-class mestizos, Mario tried to adopt the "scientific" empirical style of professional biomedicine to validate his herbal cures. For peasants and *cholos*, Nestor modified empirical practices to include more magic and ritual to administer to patients without the coldly clinical practices of biomedicine. For different classes and in their own fashion, they articulated their practice with biomedicine by adopting cures from it, by using it to sanitize ethnomedicine, and by complementing it. Their diversity of practices illustrates that Kallawaya herbalists, as well as other herbalists throughout the world, are part of a dynamic, living tradition.

Herbalists are necessary links for urban peasants in that their curing art combines traditional and modern features. They are part of the inventive aspects of culture emerging from people leaving the traditional countryside for settlement in the industrial city.

4
Shamans under Siege: Psychosocial Therapy

Although shamanism is often identified with nonindustrialized countries, there is a prevalence of shamans all over Japan today, and their popularity "lies precisely in the unsatisfactory nature of the scientific approach" (Nishimura 1987:S64).

Shamanism

The term *shamanism,* in its broadest sense, includes all efforts by healers to intercede, influence, or communicate with spirits or natural forces on behalf of the patient. In the strictest sense, shamanism is a religious phenomenon of Siberia and Inner Asia, and the word comes from the Russian Tungus *šaman* (Eliade 1987; Shirokogoroff 1935). Shamanism has also been observed in North and South America, Indonesia, Japan, Oceania, and elsewhere. Using a technique of ecstasy, shamans specialize in being able to communicate with the dead, demons, and nature spirits without becoming their instrument. Master shamans teach apprentices techniques, such as names and functions of the spirits, mythology, genealogy of the clan, ritual practices, use of vegetal drugs, and secret language. Apprentices also learn through dreams, trances, and initiatory ordeals. Among the Tungus, future shamans run away to the mountains and remain there for a week or more, feeding on animals, which they rip apart with their teeth. When they return to the village filthy and blood-stained, they babble incongruently, which indicates they have become shamans (Eliade 1987:202).

Shamans serve a great psychosocial service for members of a community. As Mircea Eliade (1987:206–7) notes, they play an essential role in the defense of the psychic integrity of the community. They war against disease, demons, and "black" magic. They defend life, health, fertility, and the world of "light" against death, disease, sterility disasters, and the world of "darkness."

The principal function of shamans is healing. Disease is attributed to something removed from the body or something inserted into the body. Latin Americans commonly complain of *susto* (fright), which is attributed to loss of *ánimo* (spirit), *ajayu* (animating fluid), or *alma* (soul)(Crandon-Malamud 1983a; Rubel 1964; Rubel et al. 1984).

72

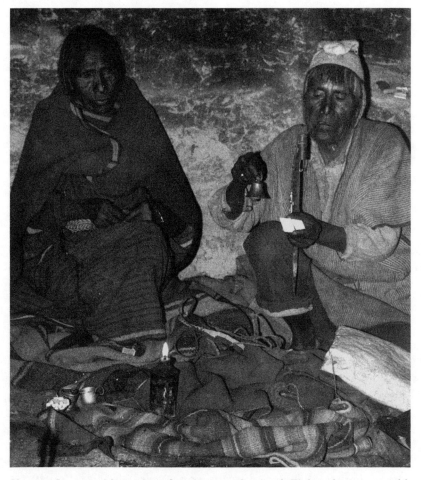

Shaman Lorenzo Mamani performing a *turka* ritual. Eighty-three years old, Lorenzo has been a principal shaman in the community of Chipaya for forty years. He is also the sacristan for the parish priest.

Latin American shamans return to the place where the person was frightened to recover the *ánimo* (Bastien 1987:42–43). Siberians attribute sickness to "rape of the soul," where the soul is stolen or wanders off. The shaman first determines which has occurred, and then begins the journey to recover it. He takes on the form of an eagle to snatch the soul from the realm of the dead (Eliade 1987:206).

When sickness is attributed to the intrusion of some object, the shaman employs sucking as a curing technique. Healers may use goat horns for cupping or a leech for drawing out blood (Sullivan 1987). Shamans frequently suck out the intruding object with their mouths, which become medical instruments that change sickening substances into something harmless. Charles Wagley (1977:191) describes Tapirape shamans of Brazil. After intoxicating themselves with great gulps of tobacco smoke, they become sick and vomit. They intermittently suck the bodies of patients and patients' vomit and accumulated saliva into their mouths. Finally they vomit it all up and search for the intrusive objects that provoked the sicknesses.

Elsewhere, shamans employ other extractive healing techniques varying from purification through washing and healing, through confession of sins, to dramatic forms of exorcisms. The exorcist casts the spirit hiding in the body out into another container, such as another animal, a tree, gourd, or medicine bundle (Sullivan 1987:232).

The essential role of shamans, however, is that of psychosocial healers: they interpret psychologically the physical experiences of illness as a reality in the social and cosmological orders. Shamans establish myths and origins of disease to provide rational and cognitive grounds for analyzing sickness and health. Cross-culturally, shamans vary in their techniques because the origins of disease are perceived differently according to the religious tradition of each culture. For example, the Semang of Kedah (Malaysia) believe that congenital diseases are attributed to the creator (Sullivan 1987:226–27). The Mondari of southern Sudan explain that certain mental illnesses are caused by Ngun Ki, the Spirit-of-the-Above (Buxton 1973:35–36).

Effectiveness of Shamanism

Mental Illnesses. Shamans contribute on a very basic level to the lives of people throughout the world and exert a tremendous influence on the treatment of mental disorders (see Kleinman 1980, 1986; Jilek 1974; Neher 1962; Nishimura 1987; Wittkower 1970). Because there is a relationship between mental illness and the cultural idiom in which symptoms are expressed (Obeyesekere 1970), shamanic rituals address this idiom and make illness meaningful to the individual and community as well as mobilize group resources, permit abreactions, and ward off cognitive and perceptual disorganization.

The popularity of shamanism in Japan for treatment of mental illness is indicated by the following studies. A psychiatrist, Nishimura (1978,) studied 300 patients in the mental ward of the public general hospital, southern Aomoro Prefecture, Japan, and found that about 80 percent had visited shamans seeking divination and, of these, 90 percent had done so before coming to the hospital for the first time. The degree of dependence on shamans varied with the illness, being close to 90 percent for schizophrenia and atypical psychosis, about 75 percent for depression, nervous conditions, and alcoholism, and 60 percent for epilepsy and organic mental disorders.

In the Aomoro study, 35 percent of the patients who had consulted shamans had been given explanations for their mental and physical disorders in terms of biomedicine, half of them being told that they had mental disorders. Thus, the recommended treatment included not only supernatural cures such as chants, prayers, and ritual offerings but also biomedicine. Patients came to the mental hospital not out of an unwavering belief in biomedicine but on the advice of shamans: biomedicine had been incorporated into shamanistic treatment as one of its subtypes (Nishimura 1987).

The following case study illustrates the interplay between shamanistic and biomedical therapies for schizophrenia in Japan (Nishimura 1987). The patient lived in the Tohoku area of Japan and was fifty-seven at the time of the study. When the patient was forty-two years old, working as a civil servant, he was plagued by a sense of isolation, auditory hallucinations, and a feeling that people were joining forces to ostracize him. He became certain that his wife had lost interest in him, was having an affair with his colleague, and wanted a divorce. He felt boxed into a corner and excluded from his family.

After he confided his condition to his wife, she told him that he was possessed by a fox and took him to a shaman to have it removed. An older male shaman, known as the "servant of the *Inari* god," prayed for him, and the patient became entranced and entered the traditional state of possession by a fox. While the shaman chanted for the fox to come out, the patient crawled around like a fox, suddenly let out a loud fox howl, jumped about, and then collapsed on the ground. He soon regained consciousness and later returned to work, but because the social situation at work had not improved, he again became depressed.

His wife wanted to take him again to a shaman, but on the advice of a superior at work, she took him to a mental hospital, where his condition grew progressively worse. He complained that he was possessed by a fox in pain and was told by the creature to say things. He was diagnosed as having a paranoid type of schizophrenia and treatment with drugs was prescribed. After a year and a half, he showed no signs of recovery and became autistic. From morning to night, he repeated, "I'm possessed by a fox in pain. . . . I'm being manipulated by a fox" (Nishimura 1987:S64).

When the patient was treated in the mental hospital with its logic of contemporary biology, the disease process became increasingly serious, beginning with the delusion of being possessed and then developing chronic symptoms. According to Nishimura, the more the patient's behavior was viewed as pathological, the more tendency it showed toward alienation from society and the more serious it became in terms of its content as a disease. The biomedical approach labeled the person a mental patient, persona non grata, and treated him in isolation from the community. The shamanistic approach considered him a member of the community and evoked the world view shared by people at the deepest level (Nishimura 1987:S64).

Diseases. For curing diseases, doctors discredit shamans by defining therapeutic efficacy as the capability of an agent, demonstrably and measurably, to alter the statistically predictable natural history of the disease (Pellegrino 1979:256). Doctors try to remove totally the cause of the disease. Equally so, shamans discredit doctors who, except for microbial diseases, cannot remove the causes of many ailments, such as cardiovascular, kidney, and liver diseases; cancer; arthritis; chronic pain; and acute respiratory infections such as grippe (see Thomas 1977).

If the underlying causes of these pathologies cannot be eliminated, how can effective treatment be assessed? Any measure of the results of medical treatment has its pitfalls, not the least of which is obvious: that diseases are self-limiting and that in some measure the body heals itself with or without ministration (Finkler 1985:118). If measuring efficacy is problematic for biomedicine, it is formidable for ethnomedicine.

Nonetheless, doctors are much more effective than shamans in curing pathological illnesses. Shamans are incapable of directly dealing with underlying biological and biochemical malfunctions. Frequently, patients do not expect to be cured by shamans: only one-third of Peruvian patients treated by shamans claimed to be cured, but the majority said that shamans were a major support during their suffering (Sharon and Joralemon 1987:9). Shamanism does not cure tuberculosis, malaria, and amebic dysentery, although it may be effective in dealing with stresses related to these and other illnesses, such as high blood pressure and heart problems.

One explanation for biological efficacy is that shamans employ medicinal plants which may not treat the targeted illness but do cure other maladies, such as worms or dietary deficiencies. For example, shamans of the Peruvian Amazon ritually use *ayahuasca*, a beverage made by concocting a malpighiaceous jungle vine, *Banisteriopsis caapi*, and the leaves of a small tree, *Psychotria viridis*, in all of their curing rituals, primarily for hallucinatory effects (Luna 1986:16), but secondarily, active ingredients effectively treat parasites and worms, common maladies in the Amazon. During all Andean rituals coca leaves are chewed, which moderate polycythemia, metabolic rates, and hypoxia.

However, the converse is also true: unexpected effects of shamanistic rituals may be negative. For example, rituals are occasions for the spread of disease when patients drink from the same ritual cup, as in Peru; share blood, as in Brazil; or vomit, which frequently occurs on taking *ayahuasca*. Shamans and rituals frequently delay patients in seeking biomedical treatment for diseases that become progressively worse (Foster 1977).

Delay of biomedical treatment is an obvious reason for simultaneous treatment by doctors and shamans. Shamans frequently recommend joint therapy (Nishimura 1987; Bastien 1989), but doctors do not. Integration of medicines flows one way for doctors and is not reciprocal, which explains why shamans object to articulation by saying, "We will lose patients!"

Because of difficulties in objectively assessing the effectiveness of shamanism, medical anthropologists focus on subjectively determined criteria that ultimately lead patients to relinquish sick roles (Finkler 1985:119). Foster and Anderson (1978) consider patient satisfaction as the final criterion. Alan Young (1977) considers Ethiopian ethnomedical practitioners effective if they enable people to deal with sickness events and provide these events with meaning. Finkler (1985:120) considers Mexican spiritualists effective if they lead patients to a subjective state of not being sick by promoting their state of well-being and satisfaction, even though they frequently fail to remove patients' subjectively perceived clinical dysfunctions.

Effectiveness of shamanistic therapy is measured by the degree to which it restores patients to their behavioral capacity and role expectations and to their subjectively perceived state of well-being (see Fabrega 1977; Finkler 1981,1985; Jilek 1974; Susser 1974). Shamanism does this *not* by the total removal of symptoms but by restructuring patients' perceptions of their dysfunctions. Shamans deal with disruptions caused by illnesses. Patients come with emotional, behavioral, and physiological symptoms, for which there may not be an organic cause and which combine to disrupt their social, religious, and economic activities. These disruptions rather than the physical symptoms are frequently the concerns of patients.

Subjective Evaluations of Shamanistic Techniques

Shamans employ certain techniques to deal with these disruptions and to restore patients to a state of well-being: bonding with patients; abrogating patients' sick role; mending social relationships; treating somatization; inducing physiological changes by meditation, trancing, and hallucinatory drugs and by theatrics, imagery, and symbols.

Bonding. One popular explanation for the effectiveness of shamanism is the bonding between the patient and the shaman. The healer-patient relationship is essential in the curing process (Anderson and Helm 1979; Fabrega and Silver 1973; Gill 1978; Haynes 1978; Pratt 1978; Finkler 1985:160). Studying shamans on the north coast of Peru, Joralemon (1984:400, 406; n.d.) and Sharon and Joralemon (1987) explain that one reason for their effectiveness is that shamans form a close relationship with clients, while also communicating their own power and authority. In the latter, they resemble doctors; but in the former, they differ. Joralemon teaches medical students at the University of Trujillo, Peru, and he invites shamans to perform curing rituals so that the students can observe shamans' techniques of bonding with their patients.

Examining what type of relationship is effective, Finkler (1985:160–61) notes that some scholars maintain that the physician's authoritative stance toward the patient enhances the patient's confidence in the physician, so that whatever the physician does is perceived to effect a cure (Parsons 1975; Siegler and Osmond 1974). Anderson and Helm (1979) and Pratt (1978) give primacy to an egalitarian relationship between patients and doctors, and Rosenberg (1979:21) contends that modern patients place their "confidence in physicians and their imputed status, and, indirectly, in that of science itself."

Scholars also differ on which elements of the doctor-patient relationship aid in fostering positive outcomes (Finkler 1985:160): that physicians with the most faith in the efficacy of their treatment achieve the best results (Benson and Epstein 1975); that communication between doctors and patients builds confidence in the curing process, especially when physicians facilitate patients' understand-

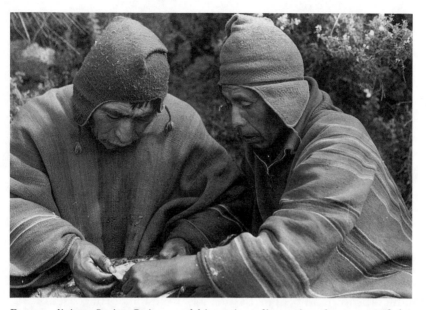

Famous diviner Sarito Quispe and his patient diagnosing the causes of the patient's illness by examining llama intestines.

ings of their impairments, of what must be done, and of the likely outcomes of therapies (Haynes 1978); that by informing patients of their conditions, physicians foster patients' compliance and cure (Inui et al. 1976); and that physicians' encouragement and instruction influence the cure (Egbert et al. 1964).

Comparison of the shaman-patient relationship to that of the physician-patient relationship is partially relevant. A better comparison would be to the psychiatrist-patient relationship. Within the psychoanalytic context, Werner (1980), Hughes (1976), and Lieban (1977) contend that by adopting the role of powerful healer, psychotherapists, like shamans, exude great authority and affect patients in a positive way (Finkler 1985:161). Smith and Glass (1977) found that therapists resembling their clients in ethnicity, age, and social level achieve more positive therapeutic results than when patients and psychotherapists are not similarly matched; other scholars have asserted that when patients select helping persons, practitioners succeed equally in assisting patients with their problems (Bergin 1971; Glasser 1977; Luborsky et al. 1975; Strupp 1980).

Studying spiritualist healers in Mexico, Finkler (1985:161) found that healing associated with religious ideologies tends to depend more upon specific healing techniques and procedures for relieving illness and less on the healer-patient relationship. Spiritualist healers are relatively impersonal, only minimally reassuring, and frequently do not share similar etiological models of illness with their patients. Similar observations are applicable to Nestor Llaves, discussed in chapter 3, who treated around forty patients a day coming from different social classes and holding different etiologies. As with Mexican spiritualist healers and Nestor Llaves, the healer-patient relationship per se is secondary to the techniques for effecting positive outcomes.

Abrogating the Sick Role. Shamans frequently perform rituals with families present that symbolically cleanse patients of their illnesses. These ritual gestures symbolically remove the patient from the role of a sick person to that of a healthy one. In Bolivia, a shaman sweeps the person from head to toe with dark llama wool, makes two bundles of the wool, places one under his cap and the other under a foot, marches to a river, and discards the illness into a stream—to afflict the lowland people (Bastien 1980). On the north coast of Peru, shamans perform *mesas,* a game board or a symbolic paradigm against which the struggle between life-taking and life-giving forces of patients takes place (Joralemon 1984:10). As shamans guide patients from the left to right sides of the *mesa,* patients pass from sickness to health. In Mexico, spiritualists cleanse their patients by lightly massaging them throughout various phases of treatment (Finkler 1985:87), symbolically removing the illness and restoring the person to health.

Shamans' cleansing of patients suggests a symbolic termination in public of the patient's sick role. According to Parsons and Fox (in Finkler 1985:162), patients assume sick roles usually for secondary gains; however, within ethnic groups, members of the family and community have different criteria for assigning people to the sick role. Among Aymaras of Bolivia, many miners are chronically sick with tuberculosis, but members of the family and community assign them to sick roles only when they are unable to work. Sometimes the inability to work is not only because of the illness, as in the case when the miners in Oruro were laid off in 1985 and were assigned sick roles and treated simultaneously by ethnomedical and biomedical practitioners for *susto* and tuberculosis. Shamans' treatment for these miners consisted largely of dealing with the social consequences of having lost their role as miners and of reintegrating them back into the work force. Doctors and nurses treated the miners for the debilitating effects of tuberculosis, enabling them to return to their communities as farmers.

Although not a concern in Bolivia, patients' somatic complaints and chronic illnesses are frequently reinforced by family and social networks as well as by biomedical practice. In the Andes, somatic complaints are reinforced as a social control mechanism. The family's sympathetic support of the patient's complaints reinforces somatization as do physicians who treat physical complaints rather than the depressive disorders with which these complaints are often associated (Katon et al. 1982, 1982a; Finkler 1985:163). Shamans in Bolivia and Peru and spiritualists in Mexico frequently fail to support patients' sick roles and tend to minimize the patients' complaints (Bastien 1980; Joralemon 1984; Finkler 1985:163). Bolivian and Peruvian shamans project these complaints on cotton balls (kintos) which are burnt and symbolically removed from the patients. These shamans conclude their rituals with meals to celebrate the return of the patients to the roles of functioning adults. The symbolic effects of cleansing, projecting, and celebrating lead patients to put an end to sick roles, particularly among patients who may be somatizing a depressive disorder.

Mending Social Relationships. Many patients visit shamans because of disrupted social relationships where they feel victimized or guilty. Common complaints are ostracism by a peer group, disagreement with employer or business partner, economic competition, marital and family difficulties, jealousy of an ex-spouse or lover, and unrequited love. In a study of sixty patients of Peruvian shamans, Sharon and Joralemon (1989; Joralemon and Sharon, n.d.) found that when asked to speculate on the cause of their condition, the most frequent responses were conflicts in marital or other love relationships (28 percent), unspecified acts of sorcery (27 percent), unknown (19 percent), environmental accident (13 percent), and 13 percent did not respond. Patients presented a blend of physical and emotional symptoms, although nearly one-third (29 percent) presented solely emotional complaints. Only 14 percent complained exclusively of physical, behavioral, or physiological symptoms. The combined effect of physical and emotional problems is the severe disruption of the individual's normal social and economic activities. Many also have experienced a personal life crisis in the recent past, attributed to bad intentions of others, effected through sorcery.

In regard to curing, patients in the Peruvian study indicated a

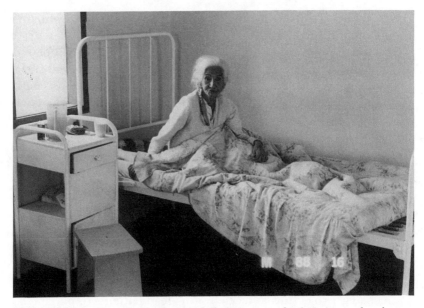

Sick Bolivian woman in the hospital. Bolivians prefer being cured at home; they believe they will die once they are taken to the hospital.

substantial drop in both the number and intensity of symptoms. These patients expressed high levels of satisfaction with the shamans, even though there were a few cases in which an unambiguous cure was reported: 37 percent said they were cured; 19 percent saw no change; and 44 percent were uncertain about the results (Sharon and Joralemon 1989:10).

Somatization. The effectiveness of shamans as physical healers is sometimes attributed to somatization, which is the process of expressing a mental condition as a disturbed bodily function. Somatization is common in nonindustrialized societies where mental illness is not recognized as such (Eisenberg 1977) and where psychological problems are not viewed as medical ones (Kleinman 1980). Somatization is also common in cultures like those of Mexico (Finkler 1985:61) and Bolivia, where psychological states are given physiological expression. Mexican spiritualists frequently treat physical disorders attributed to anger (*muina* and *coraje* or *bilis*) directly associated with interpersonal strife, especially between men and women (Finkler 1985:61). In Taiwan, Chinese frequently use somatic terminology to express emotional and mental problems, and ethnomedical practitioners treat the somatization of depression (Kleinman 1986). In the United States, hypoglycemia and chronic fatigue symptoms may be biomedicine's attempt to categorize somatized anxiety without a specific etiology (Timothy Wright, pers. com. 1992).

In Bolivia, somatization is current in cities with rural migrants, who are losing their Andean identity and suffer emotional problems of urbanized society. They lack the psychological language and cultural mechanisms of Western psychiatry to deal with emotions, so they communicate their feelings by manifesting physical symptoms, such as *mal de hígado* (bad liver) for outbursts of anger; *mal de cabeza* (headaches) for anxiety, tension, and malaise; and *dolor de espalda* (backaches) for overwork.

Frequently patients with somatization disorders are unable to be cured by doctors, who treat the somatic complaint without dealing with the emotional problems. One possible solution is for doctors to refer patients to shamans in conditions of recurrent somatic complaints of long duration for which medical attention has been sought but no physical basis for the disorder has been found. Conversely, shamans would refer patients to doctors when a physical basis for a disorder has been found which they are unable to cure. This type of collaboration can readily be done in hospitals and clinics where shamans are on the staff.

Inducing Physiological Changes. Shamans induce temporary physiological-neurological changes in patients by meditation, prayer, trance, fright, and theatrics. Recent developments in neurochemistry provide theories on how shamanistic rituals work. An early theory is that stressful treatments force the body to "snap out of disease" presumably by triggering the General Adaptation Syndrome, a hormonally mediated biological response to nonspecific stress (Selye 1956:10). In recent years, a body of biochemical data shows that physical stimulation, including acupuncture, produces analgesia by stimulating the organism to manufacture endogenous opiates (Willis et al. 1979:261; Snyder 1977; Finkler 1985:167). The stress of a traumatic ritual or morphinelike compounds, such as "endorphins," produced by the body have an analgesic effect and may be antidysphoric and antidepressant (Henry 1982; Kline 1981; Joralemon 1984:412). The release of endorphins is commonly used to explain the therapeutic effects of stress-induced altered states ranging from Salish spirit dancing (Jilek 1982) to !Kung healing (Katz 1982) and Pentecostal ritual fire handling (Kane 1982).

Shamanistic sessions might be physiologically and/or emotionally stressful to raise circulating levels of endorphins that could result in states of relative analgesia (Henry 1982:404–5) and lead to the production of altered states, such as trance. Using the Iroquois and Asclepian systems of integrating dreams into ritual, Prince (1982:418) notes that the "highly personalized threat situations are first presented in dreams and then re-enacted with the potential for intensified hormonal reactions." Shamans control the rituals so that the rush of endorphins and hormones will be experienced at the onset of the trance, and after the initial opiate rush, the affected individual will gravitate into the secondary phase of the chemical influx, resulting in a state of euphoria. This state is longer lasting because it is hormonal in nature (Henry 1982; Holt 1990:3–4). Shamans manipulate the symbols of ritual so that patients interpret these euphoric experiences as traveling to the underworld, communicating with God, or banishing monsters (Holt 1990:4). For visual representations of these states, see the paintings by Pablo Amaringo (Luna 1986:72,81,96), a Peruvian shaman who depicted visions that he saw during trance sessions.

As an alternative to the endorphin explanation, Joralemon (1984:413) has proposed that traditional curing rituals manipulate the nervous system to reestablish ergotropic/trophotropic balance. The ergotropic (energy-expanding) and trophotropic (energy-conserving) systems coordinate autonomic, somatic, and psychic functions in a balanced and reciprocal fashion (Lex 1976). The assumption is that the stimuli of ritual produce a maximal level of trophotropic tuning, pushing the body to exhaustion and permitting a reestablishment of ergotropic/trophotropic balance. Autonomic nervous system tuning is the overall physiological effect of the shaman's rituals.

These theories provide neurochemical explanations for why shamanistic rituals cause physiological effects on patients. The efficaciousness of shamanism, however, is explained not so much according to biomedical criteria but rather psychosocial criteria, such as its effectiveness as a ritually oriented symbolic system for relieving stresses (personal, social, and economic) attenuated by illness and its symptoms. Essentially, shamans are part of the management therapy group (Janzen 1978), as are doctors, which patients need. When shamans and doctors collaborate, a synergetic effect is produced which further promotes healing.

The most effective technique of shamans is their use of culturally relevant images, symbols, and theatrics to restructure the patients' perceptions of their dysfunctions and to create the imagery of mastery over the disruptions caused by illness. Their rituals are a complex interplay of physical and mental stimuli, carefully orchestrated to make the disease visible and destructible. Although part of their effectiveness is the hope of recovery instilled in the patient, which transcends biological dimensions, the other part is the reintegration of the patient into a state of well-being, which includes emotions, behavior, work, family, community, and cosmos.

Shamans employ rituals to involve patients and their families in a common symbolic sharing of experience that restores order by purification. In Africa and among American Indians and Andeans, health restoration is associated with the theme of purification (Bahr et al. 1974; Bastien 1980; Hudson 1975; Janzen 1978; Joralemon 1984). Finkler (1985:174) writes, "it is even tempting to contemplate that the imposition of order is not only a cultural imperative found in a few cultures but also a universal human imperative (Berger and Luckmann 1967; Leach 1976; A. Young 1977), perhaps even a 'human cognitive imperative defined as the innate human necessity to order sensory experience' "(Lex 1978:294).

This speculation on an innate need for order aligns with theories of personality that emphasize integration and fulfillment, but not so well with those that emphasize conflict. The integration theory emphasizes that the basic process of the personality is for a consistency in integrating diverse aspects, such as behavior and values (Allport 1937; G. Kelly 1955; Barnouw 1985:6). The fulfillment theory posits an actualizing tendency in people, involving the realization of a need for the approval of others as well as of one's self (Fromm 1955; Maslow 1968; C. Rogers 1980). The conflict theory assumes that individuals are always caught in a clash between opposing forces (Freud 1933), between which they must make compromises (Maddi 1976; Barnouw 1985:11). More in accord with conflict models of personality, shamans frequently create disorder, such as the one in Qaqachaka discussed below. Moreover, Finkler (1985:172–73) observed among spiritualist patients in Mexico and I among patients of Kallawayas, who are from many ethnic groups and classes in Bolivia, Peru, and Argentina, that there is a great deal of sociocultural and cognitive diversity. Shamanism does not resolve the contradictions but is an effective way in which people defend themselves against the contradictions, disorders, and frustrations of life by a conscious and communal process of projection, abreaction, catharsis, and sublimation.

Shamans cut through this diversity in rituals by involving the audience in dramatic theatrics. Rituals create belief in the curative powers of shamans for patients and their relatives, who in turn rein-

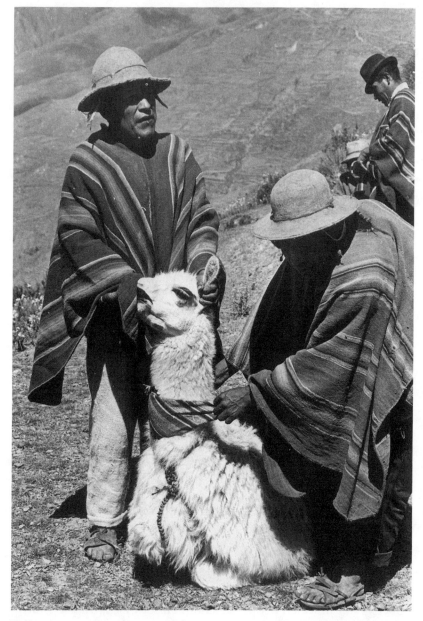

Kallawayas sacrifice a llama to Kaata earth shrines, believing that if the mountain is given a sacrificed animal it will not take humans in death.

force shamans' belief in their own power (see Levi-Strauss 1967:161–201). This triple reinforcement of belief produces a synergetic socio-psychological energy field, not much different from a good pep rally. Effectiveness is not that of efficient causality but rather of formal causality, such as found in "self-fulfilling prophecies," but with the difference that in shamanism it is a "group-fulfilling prophecy." This explains why die-hard skeptics seldom benefit from shamanism and also why other skeptics are converted in shamanistic rituals and effectively cured.

Among patients of Mexican spiritualists, Finkler (1985:174–75) observed that while symbolic manipulation by healers is crucial for perceived treatment efficacy, a patient's capacity to respond to these symbols is equally crucial and that patients unresponsive to symbolic manipulation fail totally to respond to spiritualist therapeutic intervention. Doctors and nurses face an even greater problem with many of their patients in Bolivia: the power of their healing interventions is diminished because patients don't respond to the symbolic component of the therapy. Patients (usually subconsciously) are not moved psychologically in the desired way (Timothy Wright, pers. com. 1992). In Bolivia, shamans frequently dealt with patients' unresponsiveness by carefully administering coca leaves, alcohol, and *ayahuasca* to enhance participation. In Bolivian curing rituals, participants are usually "captivated" by the imagery and symbols of the shamans, which is an indicator of shamans' skills more than a measure of participants' superstition.

The following description of a shamanistic ritual illustrates these techniques and provides a description of the imagery, symbols, and theatrics employed by shamans.

Shaman versus Nurse in Bolivia

In addition to demonstrating techniques, the following case study of a shamanistic curing ritual of the Bolivian Aymara illustrates the conflict between an auxiliary nurse and a shaman (see Bastien 1988a, 1989). Zacarias, a shaman, treated Inez, wife of Severo, the auxiliary nurse, for miscarriages. Inez was twenty-two years old and childless, which constitutes failure for Aymara women and reason for divorce. She had lost five children: Maria died after two days in a hospital; Rubén died at birth; a girl was aborted after six months, another after eight months, and finally one after two months. A doctor attributed the miscarriages to high blood pressure and prescribed medicine which did not prevent the last two. As another measure, she attended prenatal workshops on nutrition and child care, but this did not stop the miscarriages.

As an auxiliary nurse, Severo was skeptical of shamanism and opposed Zacarias in the village of Qaqachaka, Department of Oruro, Bolivia. (For ethnographic studies of Qaqachaka, see Arnold 1988, 1990, 1990a.) Severo said that Zacarias was a *farsante*, a phony. Zacarias retaliated by saying that Severo made people sick with vaccinations. This conflict curtailed the medical practice of Severo, who was classified as a foreigner and who insulated himself from the people of the community. Conservative and politically powerful, shamans have a great influence in opposing medical change. Consequently, Severo had asked for a transfer from Qaqachaka. The Ministry of Rural Health sent me to Qaqachaka to resolve this conflict. When Inez requested that a shaman cure her, I took the opportunity to persuade Severo to try this therapy. At first he refused, but slowly gave in after some persuasion.

Forty-five years old, Zacarias became a *wayt'iri* (shaman) after three theophanic events in his life—he almost died from sickness when he was young, later was struck by lightning, and nearly drowned in a torrential stream. He said that words came to him when he began reading the coca leaves. Soon after, peasants of Qaqachaka became sick in an epidemic, and he cured them with herbs and rituals.

Zacarias arrived at the house of Severo and Inez shortly before midnight on August 17, 1982, to begin a *turka* ritual, in which he employs trance as a means to call forth the complementary yet conflicting symbols of the sick person. As throughout the Andes, Zacarias read coca leaves to divine the cause of Inez's miscarriages. After several castings, he blamed them on Inez and Severo not offering rituals, on Severo having a mistress, and on sorcery. Inez became hysterical when she heard that Severo had a mistress, and they began screaming at each other.

This was a shift in that Aymara women are usually considered responsible for not bearing children. Severo now had to accept some responsibility for his wife's problems because of his improper social relations. Severo pledged his fidelity to calm Inez and to save face, but it was clear that Zacarias read from the coca what he had heard from gossip.

In comparison, one negative aspect of north-coast Peruvian shamans is that they support very basic male/female hierarchies (Donald Joralemon, pers. com. 1989). When women complain to these shamans of their husbands' infidelities, the women are told to accept this because the mistresses have slipped them love potions.

Shamans rarely blame the husbands. The same holds true for peasants when they complain about mestizos mistreating them. Peruvian shamans tell them to accept this in resignation. North coast shamans subscribe more to the cultural traditions of Catholicism and Spain with their hierarchies and subordination of woman than do the Aymara shamans of Qaqachaka, who follow Andean traditions of reciprocity between genders.

Once Zacarias had determined the causes of the miscarriages, he began the major part of the ritual and confronted powers of the underworld and the heavens. At two o'clock in the morning, Zacarias blew a whistle until he was well into a trance, a hypnotic condition similar to a somnambulistic state. Zacarias projected the voices of Saxra, Inez, and himself into a box covered with a ritual cloth. Saxra is an ambivalent symbol associated with the maternal uncle (*tio*), ancestors (*abuelos*), and the devil. Saxra represents dead relatives thought to be walking in the underground waterways. They are lonely for their live relatives and culpable for snatching babies from Inez. The effect was a trialogue emanating from the box with Zacarias as the medium. This simulated trialogue became a group argument as Inez and her husband debated with the personifications coming from the box.

Loudly and gruffly, Saxra asked: "Why have you brought me here?"

"Because you snatch babies from Inez!" Zacarias retorted.

"Why have you taken my babies?" the impersonated voice of Inez cried out.

Zacarias impersonated Inez's voice with a high pitch. Meanwhile Inez wept hysterically and screamed, "*Khitisa? Khitisa?*" ("Who are you? Who are you?").

Zacarias refereed between Inez and Saxra: "Saxra, I will not harm you. I beseech you to return her *ajayu*. I will not exchange evil." They debated back and forth for control of Inez's *ajayu*. Inez and the other participants were involved in the performance not as a representation but as an actual confrontation with Saxra.

After fifteen minutes of argument and hysteria, Zacarias calmed Inez and punished Saxra. "Saxra, you've hurt Inez and we're going to castigate you!" Zacarias slapped the top of the box with a broken cross from a rosary, a medal of Santiago, metal balls, and castanets. He asked Inez to kneel over the box, where he pounded her back, asking Saxra to return her *ajayu*. He repeated this with Severo, his ritual assistant, and me.

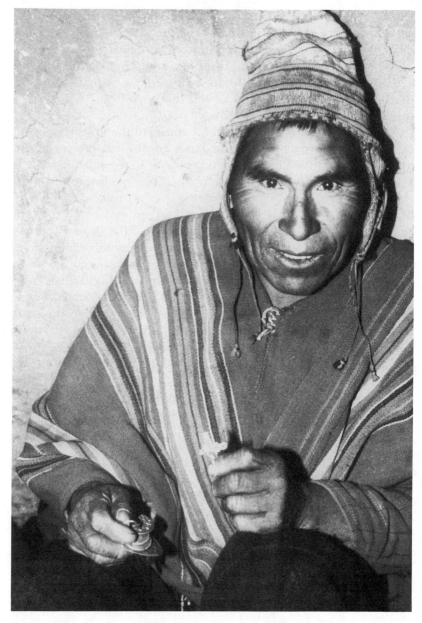

Shaman Zacarias Chiri performing ritual to cure Inez of miscarriages.

Zacarias performed a similar trialogue with the condor, Lord of the Heavens, then he impersonated the *ajayu* of Inez by crying, "Immmmmmmmmmmmmmm. . . . Immmmmmmm. . . . Immmmm."

"Jutam ajayu . . . jutam ajayu . . . Jutam ajayu!" ("Come ajayua!"), Inez called out. Inez's *ajayu* cried louder and louder.

"Makjattam ajayu!" Zacarias told her *ajayu* to enter Inez. He lightly touched Inez on the back with the metals. The *ajayu* entered her body. Zacarias also passed the sacred objects over the backs of Severo, the ritual assistant, and me. Zacarias said that everyone had been cleansed of sorcery.

Concluding, Zacarias gave each person a hard-boiled egg in a spoon. As we stood in a circle and ate the eggs, Zacarias said that we were eating all that he had done. He prayed: "These eggs are eaten in behalf of the hills for all the miracles brought forth from the earth shrines of Qaqachaka. Eat this for the health of Inez!"

The ritual began with divinations into the disruptive forces in the lives of Severo and Inez: involuntary abortions, infidelity, drunkenness, unacceptance by the community, and conflicts between Severo and the shamans of Qaqachaka. Zacarias dealt with these conflicts in a highly charged and combative fashion. Opposites were brought into battle during the ritual, with Zacarias functioning both as the fox in the chicken coop and as the farmer with the shotgun.

Nonetheless, the ritual ended with sadness and guilt. Inez felt betrayed by Severo, who got drunk the next day. Inez told us that she was five months pregnant, which worried me that the ritual might cause another miscarriage. Two years later in 1984 I ran into Severo in Challapata and asked him about Inez. He said that she had given birth to a daughter, now a year and a half old. He told me that the ritual had cured Inez and that the baby was born three months after the ritual. When I inquired how the ritual had cured her, he surprised me by saying that it had worked psychologically and by what had been later explained to him as catharsis.

Catharsis is the process of emotional discharge that relieves emotional tension (Bastien 1989:89). Unresolved emotional distress gives rise to rigid or neurotic patterns of behavior, and catharsis dissipates these patterns (Nichols and Zax 1977:206–7). Rituals provide social and cultural settings for a collective discharge that has powerful social, psychological, and biological effects, often curing people of somatic symptoms (Scheff 1979). In Inez's case, the crying relieved her of some of the grief over the death of her children, and this removed some tension, lowered her blood pressure, and resulted in the birth of a healthy baby. (This is, of course, impossible to prove because other intervening causes could have also cured her.) One objection to the cathartic theory is that after the Qaqachaka ritual,

Inez was still depressed and more anxious than ever about her husband's behavior.

Concerning the effectiveness of his shamanistic techniques, Zacarias remained authoritarian and aloof throughout the ritual, befriending neither Inez nor Severo. Zacarias symbolically brought Severo under his power when he required him to participate in more rituals. Zacarias employed ventriloquism and manipulated ritual paraphernalia to create an intensely emotional experience, shared by all. The participants were emotionally involved to the point of hysteria. In addition to catharsis, this could have triggered endogenous healing mechanisms or caused the body to snap out of the illness according to theories of neurochemistry.

Zacarias also used trance to present himself as an agent of an omnipotent spiritual force (see Koss 1975:164; Lex 1976). The abnormal psychological state of the shamanistic trance is a pathological dream state that transcends the ordinary state of consciousness, a transformation from the mundane to the sacred (Nishimura 1987:S59). Trance occurs in deep hypnosis and in hysteria, and it is likely that Inez fell into a trance, although I did not observe this. As in hypnosis, Inez followed Zacarias's suggestions and imagery without being forced to acknowledge his control or credibility. Moreover, when Zacarias directed the mediums, Inez interacted with Saxra, the condor, and him. Zacarias's method differs from spiritist ritual séances in Puerto Rico, as described by Joan Koss (1975:166), in which the cult leader is not one of the mediums, the exclusive sources of power. Nonetheless, Koss's conclusions apply to the Qaqachaka ritual in that by possession trance Zacarias controlled the participants, directed changes, and orchestrated imagery by symbols and ritual that provided a context where change could occur.

Zacarias created a cultural context in which Inez was able to deal with miscarriages, infidelity, and isolation. He provided a social context in which Severo was reprimanded and a theatrical framework where roles as husband and wife, nurse, and shaman were reenacted to better work together. Zacarias perceived the cause of Inez's miscarriages to be related to marital problems, so he dealt with them openly in the divination session. Zacarias secondarily criticized Severo for not integrating his medical practice into the belief systems of Qaqachaka, when Zacarias attributed the failed pregnancies to the fact that Severo and Inez had not fed the earth shrines.

After the ritual, Severo felt guilty and responsible for Inez's miscarriages and his lack of involvement with Zacarias and other members of the community. Either the ritual, guilt feelings, or birth of the baby caused a change, because Severo started collaborating with Zacarias. Severo and Zacarias simultaneously began treating *liquichado* patients (those whose fat has been stolen): Zacarias deals with the *kharisiri* (remover of fat) and the restoration of the "stolen fat" by diet and ritual, and Severo administers antibiotics to inhibit the tuberculin bacteria. Whereas, before the ritual, Severo discredited shamans' etiology of *liquichado* and insisted that patients come to him, he now recognizes Zacarias's role in community health. Zacarias is aware that *liquichado* patients are not permanently cured by rituals so he recognizes the need for Severo.

By 1988 Severo and Inez had three children (Denise Arnold, pers. com. 1988). Severo, Inez, and their children remain on the periphery of Qaqachaka culture and society; Severo associates with the schoolteachers from Oruro and no longer wants a transfer, Inez tends her garden and associates occasionally with mothers in the community. The people of Qaqachaka are still suspicious of biomedicine. They say that the site of the health post is a Saxra site, which the people of Qaqachaka avoid, particularly at night. They say this is why Doña Inez's children are always ill. Inez is afraid of it. Zacarias is still suspicious of the biomedical practices of Severo. The shaman's medical politics worked by legitimizing Inez's difficulties with Severo and by destroying Severo's legitimacy.

Shamans' Objections to Biomedicine

Many shamans, such as Zacarias, are resistant to biomedicine. They fear a resurgence of persecution, which was prevalent in the forties and fifties in Bolivia (but which has somewhat subsided) when the government imprisoned, fined, or shook them down for bribes, and prohibited their practice. Doctors and nurses depicted them as using fraudulent therapy that was dishonest, untruthful, and unhealthy. As masters of an old tradition, they were mocked and seen as mere cogs on the wheels of medical progress. The persecution of shamans was more severe than that of herbalists, whom doctors somewhat accepted because herbalists use empirical cures and biomedicine has a long history of herbal curing and similar origins in the Hippocratic/Galenic humoral theory. Even with the New Age craze (see Harner 1980), doctors and nurses rarely accept shamans as legitimate in Bolivia or in the United States.

Shamans fear that if they collaborate with biomedical practitioners, they will be controlled by doctors and become an inferior part of the dominant medical establishment. Zacarias, for example, maintained his autonomy over Severo and his practice by having Severo come to him to have Inez cured and by later implying that the health post is a place where Saxra dwells. Zacarias brought the nurse into his power by sociocultural beliefs, which he skillfully employs either for disease or health.

Shamans fear a power similar to what happened in the United States at the turn of the century when biomedical practitioners gained a monopoly of medical practice (Baer 1987:185–87). Doctors eliminated nonbiomedical practitioners by being the sole arbitrators of who would be certified and what would be the credentials for certification. Doctors have since determined who is legal and illegal (Starr 1982). Members of the biomedical establishment have set standards based on biomedical criteria and not on shamans' standards.

Thus, on the one hand, the possibility exists that shamans' collaboration with doctors may reduce the chances for persecution; on the other hand, the risk remains that their practices will be subordinated to biomedicine to such an extent that it would be better not to be integrated. Shamans want to know what they would gain by collaborating with doctors and nurses.

Nevertheless, shamans are adapting to biomedicine. Urban shamans prescribe pharmaceutical products and are using fewer herbal remedies. A minority refer patients to doctors, but this is uncommon. Shamans in Turco, Bolivia, participate in vaccination campaigns. Navajo medicine men bring herbs, perform rituals, and pray over patients in hospitals in Fort Defiance and Chinle, Arizona. In Swaziland, Africa, in a survey of 144 traditional healers, 98 percent of them wanted better cooperation between themselves and doctors and nurses, and 91 percent wanted training in biomedicine because they desired to increase their healing skills; but they were concerned that their lack of formal education would make "communicating with doctors" difficult (Green and Makhubu 1984). Swazi healers admired doctors for certain technical capabilities and medicines they possessed, but they felt that their ability to treat the ultimate causes of illness and to perform ceremonies, which involve cultivated relationships with spirits, were skills as important as those that doctors possessed. In Bolivia, roughly one-fifth of community health workers in the Department of Oruro are practicing shamans who accepted the post to learn about biomedicine (Oscar Velasco, pers. com. 1985).

Doctors' Opposition to Shamans

In contrast, doctors tend to be dogmatic, close-minded, and resistant to forms of healing other than biomedicine. Doctors and nurses are ignorant of how alternate medical systems work and are unable to assess their effectiveness. They judge alternate medical systems by biomedical criteria (empirical causality, laboratory tests, controlled studies, and carefully documented case studies) which depict unfavorably the psychosocial therapy of shamans. Doctors then conclude that shamanism is unscientific and therefore invalid as a medical system. Biomedical personnel lack criteria for evaluating the effectiveness of shamans.

Doctors also oppose shamans for sociocultural reasons. Upwardly mobile mestizo doctors in Latin America are prejudiced against shamanism as a form of primitivism, or a tie with their Indian ancestry. I presented a slide lecture on shamanism and herbal curing to physicians at the General Hospital in Oruro, during which one doctor violently objected that I was advocating a return to Inca medicine and stormed out of the room, shouting, "*Carajo!*"—a very strong expletive in Bolivia, used first by General Abaroa when he was asked to surrender in the War of the Pacific (1879–84) in which Bolivia lost its seacoast. The following day, another physician apologized for her colleague's behavior, saying that the upset doctor's mother is a *chola chiflera,* an urbanized Indian herbal vendor, and that this doctor was turning his back on his lower-class, Indian heritage. In the Andes, this attitude is receding due to the emergent interest in Andean nativism.

A similar reaction is reported in Africa, where African physicians, whose rise to professionalism has meant to them decolonization, Africanization of jobs, and meeting the European on equal terms, regard ethnomedical healers as an anachronism, as a throwback to a time when Europeans believed that "second best" was good enough for Africans (Warren and Green 1988). African physicians regard traditional healers as a threat to their own professionalism, and they often oppose initiatives that would result in official recognition of, or increased power of, indigenous healers. As a result "second-generation" indigenous healers adapt their methods to meet the competition and organize themselves to defend their right to practice in spite of criticism from the physicians (Last 1986). These healers are trying to get recognition from the government in order to receive a share of the salaries, supplies, and buildings that it provides.

Limiting themselves to biomedical standards, doctors criticize shamans for mistreating patients without adequate information. Shamans treat patients, many of whom are suffering intensely, with dangerous and strong drugs: San Pedro cactus, tobacco, alcohol, and coca leaves. Patients vomit violently and suffer unremittant diarrhea, which is a severe physiological stress to someone who is sick. Shamans also subject patients to long rituals that entail hallucinations and possibly terrifying visions, and emotionally ill patients may be traumatized by these visions. Shamans are unaseptic: Peruvian shamans spit sprays of perfumed water around, and people are vomiting and defecating as well as drinking from the same ritual cup.

Doctors also accuse shamans of delaying treatment of patients who are critically ill. Among shamans of the north coast of Peru and the Department of Oruro, Bolivia, this was not true: patients frequently consulted with shamans after visiting doctors and not being cured. The major problem, however, is that joint therapy results in confusing treatments so that patients frequently question the doctor's etiology, stop taking medication, and lose confidence in the doctor. This confusion of treatment is a major reason for better communication between shamans and doctors.

A still more important reason for collaboration is that shamanism is on the increase. In general, ethnomedical healers continue to be the major source of health care for about 90 percent of the world's rural population, and they are increasingly found in cities, where they treat the poor (Nishimura 1987; Buzzard 1987:31; Warren and Green 1988:4).

Education of Doctors and Shamans

Collaboration begins with dialogue among doctors, nurses, and shamans. This dialogue entails trying to understand each other's therapy and talking to one another as healers. One way is to participate in the other's healing therapy. For example, Dr. Hernan Miranda, M.D., organized a Congress of Traditional Medicine in Trujillo, July 1988, and invited Nilo Placencia, a shaman, to present a ritual for the doctors and discuss it. Nilo said that the medical association of doctors had not given him any credence in the past, so he took this opportunity seriously. He meticulously presented a shamanic ritual and carefully explained everything to the doctors. He did a convincing job and presented evidence that shamanistic healing is complex, rational, and appropriate to the local culture and environment. At the close of the congress, Miranda had to be reminded to recognize Nilo's presence, an indication of how doctors are inconsiderate of psychosocial healers (Donald Joralemon, pers. com. 1989). In similar fashion, Joan Koss invited *espiritistas* in Puerto Rico to present their cult practices to doctors and nurses.

Admittedly, shamans do not have institutionalized knowledge and practices, but there is considerable sharing of indigenous health knowledge among healers across ethnic and national boundaries (Warren and Green 1988:6) as well as a good deal of individual creativity. Doña Matilda, shaman and midwife of Oruro, has incorporated aspects of Catholicism and Bahai religions into Andean healing rituals. Shamans of the Peruvian Amazon are people who transcend the boundaries of society and go outside, where there is power. This flexibility that institutionalized medical systems like biomedicine lack permits shamanism to be very responsive and to adapt to local cultures—hence its effectiveness.

Training seminars for shamans is an approach the government health sector can take to educate them about biomedicine and incorporate them into health planning. In Swaziland, the Ministry of Health provided a series of short seminars for healers spread over five years from 1983 until 1988. The overall objective of the seminars was to establish a dialogue between healers and the ministry, focusing on priority areas of health care (diarrheal diseases, oral rehydration therapy, childhood immunization, and maternal/child health) and resulting in a two-way exchange of information on diagnosis, treatment, disease prevention, and referrals (Green and Makhubu 1984:1077). In Ghana, training sessions were more successful if they related the education specifically to indigenous healing, such as how to store and preserve herbs (Warren et al. 1982). Basic first aid is a fruitful training topic. The Ghana healers were more interested in curative than in preventive health care.

In Oruro, Bolivia, shamans wanted assistance in dealing with maladies that they were limited in curing, such as impotence, infertility, and tuberculosis. They were also interested in economic development projects, such as gardens, animal husbandry, and wells. The Ministry of Rural Health presented a one-week seminar concerning these matters in 1984. Shamans were specifically interested in psychiatric therapy. For instance, Dr. Oscar Velasco discussed with them how he had effectively used a mirror to help a woman with a disfigured face from a burn come to accept her looks and herself. He also explained how he had set up a gradual schedule for her to appear in public, supporting her throughout and helping her build confidence in herself. The shamans taught the doctors how, in the event that a patient lacks relatives or is disowned by them, to call assistants to act as relatives, adopt the person, and support him or her through the crisis.

Courses for medical students and workshops for doctors are other ways to educate biomedical personnel about shamanistic therapy. Rufino Pajjsi has presented many courses to doctors and nurses in La Paz. At the University of Trujillo, Donald Joralemon taught a course in ethnomedicine to medical students, but what impressed them most were presentations of rituals by shamans. In the Department of Oruro, Bolivia, Dr. Oscar Velasco, M.D., and I presented five-day workshops in 1983 to doctors on shamanic healing. We found that role-playing was most effective wherein an imaginary sick person was treated jointly by doctors and shamans. This usually brought laughter, criticism, and some understanding of psychosocial therapy.

Because doctors think of shamanism as simplistic and magical, ethnomedical studies can be used to provide solid evidence that shamanistic healing is complex, effective, and culturally adaptable to the local environment (Ademuwagun et al. 1979; C. Good 1987; Janzen 1978; Kleinman 1980; Leslie 1976). These studies utilize a new set of methodologies called *ethnoscience* that enables researchers to accurately record indigenous knowledge, interpret underlying structural patterns, and compare them with other medical systems. Health educators can use these studies to dispel erroneous views and simplifications about indigenous healing systems: such as, for example, that shamans attribute all diseases to spiritual causes, that they have little understanding of natural causation, and that their therapy is a closed static knowledge system.

For doctors wishing to employ shamanic techniques, Michael Harner's book *The Way of the Shaman* describes methods to acquire the experience of shamanic power to help the reader and others. Harner has practiced anthropology, shamanism, and shamanic healing for more than a quarter of a century. He markets his book as a self-help study and assumes, like Albert Schweitzer, that the shaman succeeds for the same reason that the doctor succeeds: by giving the "doctor inside a chance to go to work" (Harner 1980:174). There is a growing awareness that "physical" health and healing sometimes require more than technological treatment, that "physical" and "mental" health are closely connected, and that emotional factors play an important role in the onset, progress, and cure of illness.

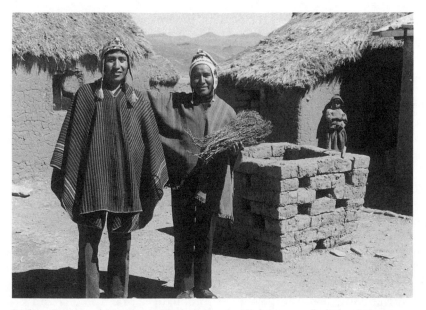

Rufino Pajjsi and his son at their home in Tiahuanaco, Bolivia. An accomplished *curandero*, Rufino educates doctors and nurses about Aymara ethnomedicine, advocating diet, herbal cures, and ritual.

Collaboration between Doctors and Shamans

Collaboration between doctors and shamans is useful if it promotes a synergetic effect via *coordination* of efforts, avoiding duplicity and counterproductive mixes of therapy. Approximately half of the average shaman's patients see doctors simultaneously, and shamans occasionally refer patients to doctors. Doctors say they don't know who the expert shamans are that they might refer patients to nor what their particular skills are. Thus, they would benefit from taking the initiative and inviting shamans to show them their skills. Well, they can't if they don't know who the shamans are.

Shamans can organize themselves into associations that monitor the training and practices of each other. In Oruro, ethnomedical practitioners have organized themselves into an association that includes midwives, shamans, and herbalists. This guild provides friendship, referrals, and information for its members, and officers of the association negotiate with members of the Ministry of Health for medical resources.

Associations of healers have proven effective in Swaziland. Before his death, King Sobhuza II called for the formation of a professional association of healers to reestablish a social control mechanism that could operate in a modernizing society (Green and Makhubu 1984:1075). Healers were motivated to form such an association because they wanted to dissociate themselves from the frauds, charlatans, and ritual murderers often linked in the public mind with indigenous healers. The king's initiative was essential because there was no tradition of formal associations or even cooperation among healers in Swaziland. Today, national associations of indigenous healers exist in a number of other African countries that have been effective in establishing a continuing dialogue between healers and governments, in the dissemination of information among and between healers, and the improvement of the quality of healing practices.

Where ministries of health in different countries encourage healers to form associations, much advantage accrues from a focus on the promotion and coordination of healing practices rather than on the control of the healers. Ethnomedical practitioners can be responsible for leadership, registration, and drawing up a code of conduct acceptable to all healers and consistent with accepted health practices. Representatives of these associations can negotiate with biomedical personnel and government officials regarding collaborative efforts in health programs. In such cases, the healers have an institution with some political representation in the government and ministry of health, which provides them with a redressive mechanism for complaints against members of the biomedical system as well as a hedge against persecution.

Some such associations have also formed alliances with scientists interested in traditional healing. The Traditional Medicine Society of Bolivia has been able to send members to international congresses because of funding from USAID. Members also participate in collaborative research with botanists, pharmacologists, and anthropologists on the pharmaceutical effects and toxicity of plants. Biomedically trained psychiatrists have contacted this society to learn more about Bolivian shamans. This association has removed some of the covert nature of shamanism and made it accessible to members of the biomedical profession.

Doctors gain when healers form associations. Associations establish criteria for membership and ethics of practice, thus providing a list of healers to refer patients to and decreasing fraud. (As with the American Medical Association, this is no guarantee of qualified healers, but there is some level of assurance.) Even though doctors are unlikely to refer patients, an association of healers can provide an educational resource that can teach doctors about synergetic healing and communication with patients. At the least, it represents an alternative healing system and provides a balancing mechanism to restore the pendulum's swing from mechanistic healing to humanistic and psychosocial healing.

Metaphorically, the image of the shaman is that of a wise, traditional person who is able to transcend the bounds of local knowledge, space, and time and deal with illnesses. In comparison, the image of the doctor is that of a scientific and dogmatic person who is immersed in a biomedical world view. A dialogue between doctors and shamans would provide doctors with an open-mindedness important to exploring the multifariousness of healing, and it would provide shamans with scientific knowledge in order to be a bit more earthly.

PART III
Mediators between Biomedicine and Ethnomedicine
COMMUNITY HEALTH WORKERS AND MIDWIVES

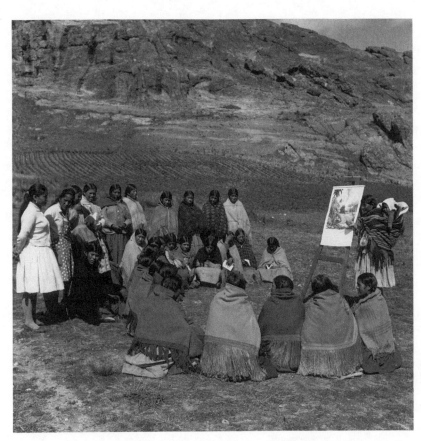

Community health worker instructing women to include vegetables in the diet at Challapata, Department of Oruro, Bolivia.

5

Community Health Workers

BRIDGING THE GAP BETWEEN BIOMEDICINE AND ETHNOMEDICINE

Community Health Workers (CHWs) serve as cultural brokers between biomedicine and ethnomedicine in certain parts of Bolivia, functioning as links between traditional practitioners within the community and doctors and nurses assigned to these communities. In developing countries, doctors and nurses frequently do not communicate effectively with peasants in rural communities. Because they are from the city, they do not speak the native languages and often do not understand ethnomedical practices. This lack of cross-cultural communication results in peasants misunderstanding biomedicine and perceiving the doctor or nurse as a threat to their ethnomedicine.

One solution is to train doctors and nurses in cross-cultural communication skills, and another is to train someone in the community to be a liaison between its members and traditional practitioners and the doctors and nurses. The role of liaison is effective if CHWs are integrated members of their communities and able to maintain their beliefs and practices in ethnomedicine. Ineffective CHWs are those who are adherents solely to the dominant medical establishment and who reject ethnomedicine, calling for ethnomedical practitioners to do likewise.

The Role of Community Health Workers: Behrhorst and World Health

The role of CHWs varies from country to country but the basic concept is an outreach program where community members become involved in their own health delivery and elect some resident to be trained in providing primary health care. One model was taken from Mao's barefoot doctor program in China, modified in Latin America by Carroll Behrhorst (1972, 1974, 1975, 1983) in Chimaltenango, Guatemala, and finally adopted and recommended by the World Health Organization at Alma-Ata in 1978 (Newell 1975; WHO and UNICEF 1978). In Latin America the term *promotor de salud* is used to designate community health workers, and I translate this as health promoter or simply promoter.

Chimaltenango Model. Carroll Behrhorst's CHW program among the Cakchiquel Indians of Guatemala has been a model for similar projects in Bolivia and other parts of the world (see Bastien 1990:281–87; Crandon-Malamud 1983; Glittenberg 1974; Heggenhougen 1976; Phillips 1990:167–77; Steltzer 1983). In 1962, Behrhorst left a medical practice in Kansas and went to Chimaltenango, where he worked as a doctor for nineteen years, establishing one of the most innovative community health worker projects in the world. In a survey of twelve community health projects in Latin America in 1977, Dr. Fritz Muller of Utrecht, Holland, found that CHWs in Chimaltenango were the best trained and most effective health workers he had observed (Behrhorst 1983:xix).

Behrhorst (1983:xi–xii) believed that before health can supplant disease among the rural poor of the world, the following problems must be tackled aggressively in this order:

1. Social and economic injustice
2. Land tenure
3. Agricultural production and marketing
4. Population control
5. Malnutrition
6. Health training
7. Curative medicine

Behrhorst listed curative medicine last, which he considered first at a clinic in 1962 when he treated 125 patients the first day. After seeing the same patients returning months later with the same ailments, he realized that no matter how many times he treated them, they would never be healthy until drastic changes were made in their villages.

The key to realizing these priorities in Guatemala was the training of responsible Indians to be health promoters (CHWs). After a certain amount of inexpensive training, health promoters treated the most common afflictions just as well as a university-trained doctor. They responded better than doctors to the customs of the people and were invaluable in implementing public-health projects and the development of other needed community services (Behrhorst 1983:xviii). They became involved in land reform and in soliciting legal support against land encroachment.

By 1980 CHWs had increased to more than seventy individuals from fifty communities. Health promoters were required to be carefully selected and continuously trained and supervised in practical medicine. At first, candidates were recommended by local priests or Peace Corps volunteers, but later, a community participatory approach was adopted to select them. Members of the community set up a community betterment committee, which included a health committee. Then the health committee selected the person to be trained. Promoters represented their communities, and communities were responsible for them and could discipline them, recommending their renewal or dismissal.

Training was demonstrative and continuous: health promoters came once a week to Chimaltenango and spent a day at the hospital, making the rounds with a doctor or supervisor. Health promoters saw patients and learned about their problems as well as how these problems could be treated or prevented in their home villages. They discussed symptoms rather than diseases, since symptoms have more meaning to villagers than disease entities. Seeing a patient with an ailment and discussing it provided a more valuable teaching experience than hours of lectures.

Before health promoters were allowed to dispense medicines and give injections, they had to attend these sessions for one year. They were required to pass periodic exams in which they described what they observed in a patient, what could be done for the ailment, and what needed to be done in the patient's home to prevent a recurrence of the problem. The majority of health promoters attended these weekly sessions, some for ten years, and successfully passed the exams. Of importance, a supervisor regularly visited health promoters on the job to support, consult with, and advise them. The supervisor was Carlos Xoquic, a Cakchiquel Indian and highly respected elder who had been a promoter for many years. Carlos had complete charge of the CHW program, and he consulted a doctor, or another professional, only when, in his opinion, the problem warranted it (Behrhorst 1983:xix).

In analysis, the success of the Chimaltenango CHW project was due to its simplicity in using indigenous resources (community responsibility and leadership regarding health and land reform), in training and supervising health promoters continuously and periodically with practical and culturally applicable lessons, in the lack of a bureaucracy, and in the embedment of the program in land reform and legal aid to facilitate access to land.

Unfortunately, the program's success in land reform led to some problems. Because CHW programs in Chimaltenango and other parts of Latin America helped create leaders in peasant communities, some have been accused of training revolutionary leaders. In Guatemala, the health promoter program became a target by which the military sought to destroy indigenous leadership in an effort to wipe out present and potential opposition to military control and oppression. In the Ayacucho area of Peru, the military also suppressed CHWs for allegedly supporting terrorism. In Bolivia, national leaders did not actively support CHW programs from 1980 until 1985 for fear that CHWs would become terrorists. As a result, CHW programs in these countries have become less independent of the dominant medical establishment and government, being subjected to more bureaucracy and control.

Sensitive to these political issues, the planners of WHO at Alma-Ata in 1978 modified Behrhorst's model. They mostly avoided references to land reform and said nothing about legal support against land encroachment. Neither did they remark on the lack of bureaucratic structure nor the ongoing clinical education received by Chimaltenango promoters that made Behrhorst's model work so well (Libbet Crandon-Malamud, pers. com. 1990). Still, in an innovative way, these planners established the need for CHWs throughout the world and supported Behrhorst's (1983:xvii) message of the myth of the "indispensable doctor."

According to the World Health Organization, one advantage of CHWs is that in developing countries with a shortage of doctors and nurses, CHWs can provide health care for masses of people living in rural areas and urban slums. As Behrhorst (1983:xviii) observed, in developed countries people erroneously believe that a doctor is indispensable and that only a medical doctor with a degree acquired after long academic training is competent to cure even minor ailments. Even in industrialized countries the vast majority of patients are in no real need of a sophisticated doctor. In short, the world needs inexpensively trained, reasonably affordable, and locally available health workers for villages, communities, and cities as alternatives to nurses and doctors.

Since Chimaltenango and Alma-Ata, CHWs have begun to treat patients in rural communities throughout the world, some more successfully than others. In Nigeria, for example, Ekunwe (1984) writes that doctors are unevenly distributed and overspecialized, so they have trained CHWs who function as "physician extenders," treating patients whose needs are simple and referring difficult cases (5–10 percent) to the doctor. They are educated from ten to eighteen months in health needs of their communities. Unfortunately, they have not been fully utilized and are only allowed to make cursory home visits (Iyun 1989:937). Worldwide, national-level CHW programs have received pluses and minuses (Berman et al. 1987; Wood 1990:123).

Community Health Workers in Asia. In Korea, Kim (1987) writes that 2,000 community health practitioners are involved in the delivery of primary care in rural areas. These practitioners are nurses and/or midwives who have completed a six-month course and are preferably selected by the communities where they serve. They are responsible for maintaining a primary health post, organizing community development, and supervising village health volunteers. They are reported to have performed well and been accepted by the people. Disadvantages of CHWs in Korea are the costs involved in training and a high turnover rate of participants.

Community health workers are sometimes selected for their political connections rather than their dedication to health issues. In India, for example, Mahadevappa (1984) writes that if the selection of the candidate is left up to the community, they will frequently select someone who is a distant relative of the local political leader or even just a political follower. Selection of skilled candidates is the exception rather than the rule. Mahadevappa concludes that in India, with only 1.8 percent of the GNP being spent on health, the cost involved in the training and retraining of CHWs is too high. Moreover, at a time when quackery is rampant in India, it is naive to overlook the possibility of CHWs attempting to function as private medical practitioners.

Maori Community Health Workers. Among the Maori people of New Zealand, CHWs satisfy a strongly felt need by partially bridging the gap separating their people from full utilization of existing biomedical services (Wood 1990:133–34). CHWs have formed their own association, which is part of a culturally sensitive and community-based health care, popular alongside other nationalist movements such as sweeping political activism, language acquisition programs, restoration of long-neglected *marae* (traditional Maori ceremonial centers), and renewed pride in traditional Maori art forms and legends. Even more important, CHWs have linked good health status with other development issues, such as the rejection of alcohol and tobacco. They have influenced Maori political consciousness far in excess of whatever they may have done to lower morbidity and mortality rates (Wood 1990:134).

The success of Maori female CHWs has been limited by the

marginalization imposed on them by their dependence on the good-will of male doctors for training and support. These doctors see female CHWs as less worthy and are unwilling to support them adequately. Maori CHWs not only lack a well-defined sphere of activity but also their health-care tasks have been relatively few (Wood 1990:134). Likewise in Bolivia, female CHWs received less support from doctors than male CHWs. Many women aspired to be CHWs in Bolivia, but they quit after some time because of lack of support, difficulty of traveling alone, and domestic responsibilities. Solutions are to define their responsibilities with doctors, to reward women CHWs with role status, to see that they are accompanied on journeys, and to have other members of the community assume their domestic responsibilities.

Morbidity and Mortality. Berman, Gwatkin, and Burger (1987:457) argue that it has yet to be demonstrated that CHWs have reduced morbidity and mortality in any substantial way. Statistical decreases in morbidity and mortality are more a result of general improvement in the standard of living rather than interventions by CHWs. They conclude that existing CHW programs have low costs but also low effectiveness.

In response, it is difficult to evaluate the effect of CHW programs on morbidity and mortality because they are relatively new, have been marginally accepted by politicians and doctors, and only recently are gaining respect. In many places, CHWs have contributed significantly to public-health measures. They have also fulfilled important objectives of primary health care to have members of the community participate in health care and to incorporate ethnomedical practitioners. Many CHWs are practitioners of ethnomedicine, and thus they bridge the gap between alternative medicines.

Another reason why morbidity and mortality statistics are not effective evaluation measures for CHWs and ethnomedical practitioners is that often these practitioners have other objectives besides removing illness and preventing death, such as psychosocial support, redressing grievances, and community solidarity. In Guatemala and Bolivia, CHWs are significant forces in economic development. Corinne Wood (1990:134) points out that even though Maori CHWs may not lower morbidity and mortality, their "loving hands" movement has filled and continues to fill a serious need.

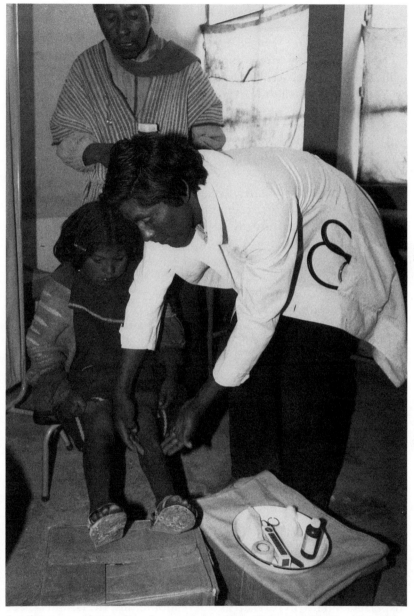

Auxiliary nurse Santos Paredes treating a young Chipaya girl with scabies. The president of the health committee looks on. Chipayas accepted biomedicine in 1970.

Health Needs and Community Health Workers in Bolivia

In Bolivia, promoter projects have been attempted, some with more success than others, providing lessons for adaptation to the Chimaltenango model and WHO directives. These projects provide attempts to train health workers selected by the community, to provide ongoing supervision while avoiding unnecessary bureaucracy, and to bridge the gap between bio- and ethnomedicine. "Attempt" is used because CHW projects in Bolivia and elsewhere are greatly influenced by the political economy and existing health problems (Gish 1979; Morgan 1987).

One problem of rural health care in Bolivia is the use of auxiliary nurses (*enfermerías auxiliares*) in many and distant communities. Auxiliary nurses constitute the principal biomedical personnel throughout rural Bolivia, although there are a limited number of doctors in hospitals. Auxiliary nurses are little trained (six months to a year after secondary school), poorly paid ($50 a month in 1985), supervised in a disciplinary fashion, and subject to bureaucratic control (biweekly reports to administrators in the cities of the departments). Many live apart from their families in other communities so that time is spent traveling back and forth to hand in reports, receive their salaries, and visit their families. Many nurses do not speak Aymara and Quechua languages and cannot communicate cross-culturally with peasants, the majority of whom speak these languages, especially the women and children.

Although efforts are being made to improve education for nurses, such as the school for auxiliary nurses in Cochabamba, the Bolivian Ministry of Rural Health is unable to increase their salaries or finance *items* (health-post positions) for the myriad of rural communities throughout Bolivia. Bolivia covers an area of 679,619 square miles and, in 1987, had an estimated population of 6.7 million, a population density of 10.8 people per square mile and a population growth rate of 2.6 percent per annum (Project Identification Document 1988). Forty-three percent of the population are less than fifteen years old. Forty-eight percent of the population live in localities of more than 2,000 inhabitants. The other 52 percent are widely dispersed and live in rural areas where mountains, rivers, and lack of roads make travel difficult.

Mortality rates in Bolivia point to the need for better trained and additional health personnel. According to the Project Identification

Document (1988), the maternal mortality rate is estimated at 48 per 10,000 live births, the highest in Latin America. This and other mortality rates are probably higher since Bolivian statistics are unreliable. Infection, hemorrhage, and induced abortion are the principal causes of maternal mortality. Malnutrition and anemia are important associated causes of mortality. The total fertility rate is high, with a national average of 6.1 children per woman. Peasant women are at a disadvantage due to low literacy rates, limited access to money, and male domination. Infant mortality rates (number of deaths within the first year out of every 1,000 born) range from 97 to 134 in urban areas and 120 to 210 in rural areas. The rate for the nonsalaried agricultural families is from 245 to 333 in certain areas. The major reported causes of infant and child mortality are (1) acute diarrheal infections, (2) acute respiratory infections, (3) perinatal infections, and (4) infections that would be preventable by immunization. Respiratory infections most heavily affect children under one year old, among whom the risk of death from all causes is seven times as high as that among children one-to-four-years old (PID 1988).

Bolivia educates many doctors but 70 percent emigrate to other countries (*Evaluación* . . . 1978:305). In cities, there is an average of one doctor for every 1,000 Bolivians, as compared to one for every 7,000 peasants in the countryside. Doctors rarely speak the Aymara and Quechua languages, consider peasants inferior, and are neither trained nor committed to work in rural areas, being required and paid by the MPSSP (Ministerio de Previsión Social y Salud Pública) to work a year (*año de provincia*) in rural areas after graduation (see Bastien 1987a, 1988).

The MPSSP provides primary health care to rural communities with health posts (*postas sanitarias*) staffed with auxiliary nurses, an average of one per 1,500 peasants. Providing practical and ongoing training in rural health and support for auxiliary nurses, must come from the MPSSP and the community: supervisors need to be less bureaucratic and more supportive, and communities need to form health committees and elect and support CHWs. In some parts of Bolivia, CHWs have formed outreach programs extending to communities distant from the health posts. The role of CHWs in Bolivia is similar to that of village health volunteers in Korea, who assist the community health practitioners by home visiting, providing basic medicine, giving advice on health matters, referring cases to primary health posts, and collecting data.

Unsuccessful Community Health Workers Projects in Bolivia

Achacachi. In Bolivia, CHW projects were unsuccessful in Achacachi and Montero. Achacachi is an important peasant center near Lake Titicaca, about 100 km west of La Paz (see Albo 1979). A Maryknoll priest with nursing and public health degrees, Joe Picardi started the Achacachi project in 1975. Health promoters supposedly motivated by love of neighbor and by the welfare of the community worked without salary. Initial enthusiasm was high, with 100 promoters in 1975, but which ebbed to 16 in 1980. They were trained in a series of one-week courses which qualified them to pass through three levels (Joe Picardi, pers. com. 1981). Candidates for the first level were required to own land, know how to read and write, and be nominated by the community. They were taught to build latrines and vaccinate children in immunization programs. After they returned to their villages and did the above, they were then qualified for the second level, where they were taught to install water filters and put chimneys on houses so the smoke from cooking fires could escape. In similar fashion, if they installed the filters and chimneys, they could return for the third level, where they were taught problem-oriented charting. Each promoter was trained to keep accurate information concerning symptoms and treatment. Doctors and nurses in Achacachi checked these reports monthly. Promoters also formed mothers' clubs in their communities and thus encouraged links with *Caritas*.

The Catholic Relief Agency (*Caritas*) supports 3,000 mothers' clubs throughout Bolivia by donating surplus food from the United States government to mothers who attend weekly meetings. The association of CHWs with mothers' clubs has some disadvantages. Although mothers' clubs serve as focal points for educating women in Bolivia, they also discriminate against nonchildbearing women; create dependency on free food; and in a very limited manner, support family planning by the rhythm method, being supervised by Catholic charity.

In comparison to Chimaltenango, supervision, practice, and ongoing education were also the bases of the Achacachi CHW program. Although the Chimaltenango program depended greatly on Behrhorst, the Achacachi program depended exclusively on Joe Picardi, and after he left Bolivia in 1980 the program stopped in 1981. Major differences were that Behrhorst placed Carlos Xoquic, a promoter, in charge and that Picardi overemphasized biomedicine. Picardi did not permit ethnomedical practitioners to become health promoters and discouraged collaboration with them. As a result, promoters often opposed herbalists and ritualists, who perceived their authority to be threatened. Traditional practitioners were, and still are, important leaders of these communities, and they refused to acknowledge the role of health promoters. Few health promoters were able to establish a role in their communities even though they were elected by the members. Another reason for the project's demise was that promoters saw it as a means of supplementing their income, and when they found out there was no money in it, they quit. In short, Achacachi CHWs were not integrated into their communities or the MPSSP, which was also discouraged by the military government of President García Meza from training health workers in Achacachi because it is a community near Peru where the terrorist group *Sendero Luminoso* (Shining Path) is active.

Montero. Poorly planned and mismanaged, the CHW project in Montero, Department of Santa Cruz, began in 1975 with a budget of $381,900 under the Methodist Church, USAID, and MPSSP. The grant was increased to $927,500 in 1976. For evaluation of the Montero CHWs, see Crandon-Malamud (1977, 1983), Donahue (1981), and Kraljevic (1977, 1978).

This project chose to structure the delivery system on the already existing rural educational infrastructure (Donahue 1981:175–76): larger communities (nuclear communities) often had schools with all primary grades, which served satellite communities with only a few primary grades. The nuclear communities (eight) had either a hospital or medical post, and the satellite communities (thirty-one) had no health facilities. The nuclear community had an auxiliary nurse "I" who supervised health promoters and health committees in the satellite communities. Stationed at the district hospital, auxiliary nurse "II" supervised activities of auxiliary nurse "I." Finally, an extension team of nine health advisors and a data-collection team would intervene at the nuclear and satellite levels to do research and support the auxiliary nurses and health promoters.

During 1976, sixty-eight auxiliary nurses were trained in three six-month courses. The outreach team and auxiliary nurses contacted the satellite communities to form health committees. They chose the first group of seventeen health promoters during the agricultural off-season, the majority of whom were married men who were able to return to their communities for planting. They chose the second group during planting season; the candidates were mostly young unmarried men and women without major agricultural responsibilities. By January 1978, promoters in some communities had not been paid. The situation was most critical in those communities that had older, unmarried promoters who could not afford to work without remuneration. Younger promoters who had not been paid were being supported by their parents (Donahue 1981:180–81). The project was capital intensive, which meant that when the funds ran out, health promoters were left poor and disillusioned.

Other problems arose: conflicts occurred between the existing public health system and the community-based CHW program. Auxiliary nurses "II" observed that they had no difficulties where there were no health facilities and where the people saw the need for health care and were more open to the idea of preventive medicine, but in areas with health facilities, patron-client relationships affected the choice of health committee members and promoters, which polarized community members (Crandon-Malamud 1977:4). Some communities were stratified into locals and immigrants— often wealthier migrants, who because of their economic position in the community were "elected" to the health committees (Kraljevic 1978). In one instance, Kraljevic observed that community elites were divided on the election of a young woman as health promoter whose father had advanced her candidacy to enhance his family's prestige at the expense of other elite family interests in the community.

Another conflict arose when local leaders of communities selected for the project offered stiff resistance to a government health program in their communities (Donahue 1981:190–91). Simply put, project leaders and educators had not previously prepared the community leaders and members. Other communities were selected, but these diverged from several of the selection criteria, such as Antofogasta, which had a hospital, inaccessible satellite communities, and a highly transient population. As a result, the project served not only areas already with health care but also a small number of people: the total population of the pilot communities was only 15,000, or half of what was originally planned.

A fundamental problem of the Montero project was the shifting social boundaries of many of the communities in the Santa Cruz area (Donahue 1981:184). Traditional definitions of community groupings based on common name, legal status, and other geopolitical descriptors were often misleading, especially in areas of intense emigration from Aymara and Quechua regions with distinctly Andean patterns of social organization. This misunderstanding by planners led to many intra- and intercommunity conflicts because the project was frequently misaligned with actual political, cultural, and social groupings.

Failures were evident from the support side. The Ministry of Health (MPSSP) had difficulty filling counterpart positions that were necessary to facilitate the flow of information and services among the national, regional, and local offices. Several advisor positions under the responsibility of USAID were also vacant during the start-up period (Donahue 1981:190). The weakest link in the program was the auxiliary nurse "I," who played a key role in the interfaces of the project, between the MPSSP, the hospital, health committees, health promoters, and residents of each community. Because selection criteria required a high school diploma, the majority of these nurses were young men and women. This excluded the older, more mature and respected members of the community. Furthermore, the roles of nurses and promoters overlapped: where the project envisioned that the auxiliary nurse would provide medical support services and supervise the promoters, members of the community viewed the nurses as more qualified and of greater status (Donahue 1981:188).

By 1985, the Montero project was abandoned. It was rumored that USAID pulled out in opposition to President García Meza (Libbet Crandon-Malamud, pers. com. 1990), but more likely causes were disappointing results and lack of funds. This failure made many peasants and health workers resistant to future CHW programs in Bolivia. The experiences at Achacachi and Montero provided lessons on the essentials for a successful CHW program: an understanding of indigenous cooperation and interaction is an important first step; health promoters need to be elected and supported by their communities since the government cannot afford to pay their salaries; promoters must work with traditional medical practitioners, and they must involve community members in an integrated health program that includes access to land, agricultural production, and marketing, as Behrhorst (1974) pointed out (Donahue 1981:193).

Recommendations. In planning health programs for indigenous communities, whether in Bolivia or other parts of the world, a cooperative strategy is the most effective. In Bolivia, for example, Aymara and Quechua communities have long traditions of mutual assistance and reciprocity. When government projects, such as in Montero, fail to recognize the parameters of indigenous cooperation and interaction, they stimulate intercommunity rivalries and fragmentation (Buechler and Buechler 1971; Bastien 1978). If rural health programs in Andean countries ignore the social and cultural parameters of intra- and intercommunity interaction, support for a cooperative venture is unlikely.

Caution is required in the choice of criteria for defining catchment areas to be served by health promoters and auxiliary nurses. The presence of a school, *corregidor,* plaza, or *junta communal* may reflect more recent divisions introduced into the community and not the traditional *ayllu* health-care system (Donahue 1981:193). Throughout the Andes, *ayllus* are distinguishable groups whose solidarity is formed by religious and territorial ties *(llahta ayllu),* by permanent claim to land and lineage *(jatun ayllu),* by affinal ties *(masi ayllu),* and by work *(mit'a ayllu).*The *ayllu* may not be contiguous with any one political boundary, but may incorporate several such "communities" into the traditional patterns of reciprocity and communal activity. Indeed, these bonds may include migrants from the communities in nearby cities.

A problem with the Achacachi program was the restructuring of social relations of the CHWs with members, leaders, and ethnomedical practitioners of the community and with auxiliary nurses and doctors supervising primary health care for these communities. CHWs were trained and expected to engage in certain activities by the project directors, who were under the MPSSP and who advocated biomedicine, and at the same time they were elected and supported by members of the community, who often had different expectations, which varied from getting free food to taking the preliminary steps toward getting a hospital. Hence, CHWs found themselves in a double bind, facing conflicting expectations, which sabotaged the very legitimacy they needed to get the job done.

One way to avoid this problem is to have doctors and nurses discuss health needs with members of the community as well as the ways CHWs would deal with these concerns. Health workers need to orient their policies to the values of the people (E. Rogers 1983:318). This is difficult because doctors and nurses tend to be directive- and establishment-oriented rather than community- and culture-oriented. Auxiliary nurses and doctors also need to be educated about their working relationship with CHWs.

CHWs in Achacachi and Montero had an intermediate role between doctors and nurses of the Ministry of Health and leaders and ethnomedical practitioners of the communities. Not rooted in either camp, their role was ambivalent, and they had to be ambidextrous, adapting to whatever side was most demanding. This led to frustration and lack of authority. It was like being a civil defense officer, adjunct professor, or voluntary cop in the United States, with little authority or benefits from the community and the institution. Their role was not consistent with other political roles in the community and the Ministry of Health. It became questionable whether the role of CHWs could accommodate two different social and cultural organizations or whether a role should be designed to fit within the biomedical system and Andean community. The functional relationship between roles in the Ministry of Health is basically one of hierarchy, authority, and control, all covered by an inefficient bureaucracy. Consequently, auxiliary nurses, who are the major personnel in the rural health delivery system, are relatively ineffective.

Cultural Adaptation: Community Health Workers in Oruro

Project Concern Oruro (PCO) and the Ministry of Rural Health, Oruro (MRHO), attempted to adapt the role of CHWs to Andean political roles. MRHO is a branch of the MPSSP, the governmental health program for Bolivia. PCO is an operation of Project Concern International, a private voluntary organization with headquarters in San Diego, California. Prior to 1982, Project Concern had been unsuccessful in Cobija, a jungle town in Bolivia. Gregory Rake and Angela Lutena redesigned Project Concern's operations in Bolivia and are responsible for the success of the Oruro project. Rake has a master's degree in medical anthropology from Kenyon College, and Lutena has R.N., M.N., and M.P.H. degrees as well as years of experience working as a rural health educator. Adapting Behrhorst's ideas to Bolivia, Rake and Lutena advocated the articulation of traditional and modern medicine. They also worked closely with MRHO and did not create another departmental structure for the program.

Directed by doctors and favoring biomedicine, Project Concern International (PCI) provided little support to Rake and Lutena until 1985, when USAID favorably evaluated them, began funding them, and used the Oruro CHW project as a model for its training of health promoters and the integration of traditional medicine. Burned out from his efforts with PCI, Rake went to work with the Medical Assistance Program (MAP) in Ecuador in 1985. This conflict between Project Concern Oruro and Project Concern International illustrates the tensions that exist for bilateral agencies with regional versus international directors and the overseas staff versus the home staff. Administrators in donor countries complain about the field staff which is "causing difficulties" by refusing or failing to carry out programs as originally envisioned in the project agreement. And field staff members accuse head office people of being out of touch with a particular culture and its environment (Mosley 1987:53–54).

Breakdowns in understanding between home and abroad increase when projects—such as the integration of bio- and ethnomedicine—rely less on technical design and more on flexibility, cultural knowledge, appropriateness, and cross-cultural communication skills. Bureaucrats want projects to follow the plan and not be subject to unexpected adjustments. As a result, culturally sensitive health issues at the regional level are unlikely to be resolved at the international level with universally agreed-upon biomedical health policies. Regional directors need flexibility and autonomy in adapting CHW programs and primary health care to highly variable political roles and social organizations within the community.

Beginning in 1982, Rake and Lutena trained seventy health promoters in three one-week courses. See Bastien (1987:90–91) for a description of their training and activities in the community. By 1988, sixty-four were still working, and twenty seven (39 percent) had been health promoters for six years. They functioned in their communities as health workers, agents of change, and mediators between ethno- and biomedicine. They maintained rudimentary dispensaries and treated diarrhea, acute respiratory infections, parasites, and scabies in addition to administering first aid for injuries. They had built gardens, ovens, and latrines and had formed mothers' clubs and educated members of the community in public health. Many had become actively involved in community and rural development.

Ideally, the community was to play as much a supervisory role for health promoters as Project Concern and the Ministry of Health. Before any community elected a promoter, its members attended a series of talks about preventive medicine and public health being their responsibility. Only after all members of the community were willing to participate in these health matters were they allowed to elect a promoter. The core idea was that health is not something given; it requires a collaborative effort by all members of the community. The promoter represents efforts of community members, and is effective to the degree that they participate in health matters. This is based on the Andean pattern of a leader being one who represents the collaborative efforts of the group.

Members of the community elect a qualified promoter for three years. The qualifications are that the man or woman be a literate adult, living in the community most of the year and willing to work without salary toward improving the health of the community. Members of the community can vote to have a CHW removed from office, an action that is reviewed and can be vetoed by the supervisors. Removal of a CHW happened several times, once because the promoter used the position for evangelizing and twice because promoters were charging excessive fees. More unilaterally, doctor and nurse supervisors can remove a CHW from office without approval of the community. Although consent of the community is not needed, Rake and Lutena always consulted with members of the health committee and community before dismissing a promoter, which was usually for inactivity.

At first, some health promoters were elected in puppet elections, but this was later avoided by requiring signatures of all members of the community as well as supervision of the election by the auxiliary nurse. In other instances, health promoters who were elected by blocks of proselytizing Protestants (Nazarenes, Seventh-Day Adventists, Jevohah's Witnesses) caused division in the communities, opposed traditional practitioners, and were resistant to ethnomedicine. As an example, Guillermo was a promoter in the village of Cotuto, Province Abaroa, for two years. After his election in 1982, Guillermo became a rabid evangelist and preached against ethnomedicine and ritual practices as the work of Satan. Catholics and traditionalists opposed him and members of his church. Implicitly, his activity suggested that evangelism and the role of health promoter were tied together. The conflict increased until Guillermo left the village in 1984. After that, Gregory Rake established the policy that health promoters be discouraged from using this role to change people's beliefs or to promote Christian religions.

The Politics: Leadership Roles

The role of CHW also came into conflict with that of the auxiliary nurse mainly because health promoters and nurses did not understand one another's role in the community and vied for medical control. Jorge was CHW of Riobamba, Province Sur Carangas, and for six months had been in conflict with the nurse, who had publicly criticized him for giving injections, practicing veterinary medicine, and overcharging for medicines. Health promoters are required to charge standard fees for medicines, which are paid to the MRHO. In retaliation, Jorge complained that the nurse didn't care for the sick of Riobamba and frequently traveled to Oruro. Typical of feuds, both of them sought support from political officials and members of the community. The *alcaldes escolares* (supervisors of schools) and *alcaldes de caminos* (supervisors of roads) sided with the promoter. The *corregidor* (sheriff) supported the auxiliary nurse because he was her *compadre* (ritual kin). The promoter lived in an outlying village and its members supported him; the auxiliary nurse worked in the community of Riobamba whose members supported her.

Angela Lutena and Oscar Velasco met with the leaders of Riobamba to resolve this conflict. A Bolivian doctor employed by the Ministry of Health, Velasco supervised promoters and was in charge of the integration of ethnomedicine. Before joining the project, he had spent ten years working in rural communities, using ethnomedicine whenever possible. The auxiliary nurse complained to Lutena and Velasco that she would go to vaccinate members of the promoter's village and nobody would be there; Jorge replied that she had not advised him beforehand, which she interpreted as needing his permission. The promoter, an elder of fifty years, with a long record of fulfilling *cargos* (civic responsibilities), said that the auxiliary nurse, a woman of twenty-four years, supervised him in a humiliating manner. They never settled the dispute and both were temporarily suspended. Later, some members of the community asked that the auxiliary nurse be reinstated, which she was, but she soon left to work in another community. Jorge continued to practice medicine, human and veterinary.

This example illustrates a breakdown in social and working relationships between personnel at different levels of the health system bureaucracy. To prevent similar problems, directors of the Oruro project now invite auxiliary nurses and doctors to participate in training sessions for health promoters. The relationships between health promoters and auxiliary nurses and doctors are key factors in the success of this outreach program.

Contrary to the case in Riobamba, auxiliary nurse Nelly Gutiérrez and promoter Clemente Montero established a highly compatible relationship in the community of Ancacato. To avoid conflict, Rake and Velasco had adopted a policy not to elect promoters in communities where nurses were working, but because the people of Ancacato petitioned to have a promoter, an exception was made. Initially, Nelly and Clemente disagreed over responsibilities, but soon agreed on how they could collaborate. At present, Clemente frequently travels with Nelly, since traveling alone is difficult for a woman in the Andes. Clemente's son also accompanies them to avoid any criticism. In one instance, they traveled six hours to deliver a baby. The baby was born before they got there, but the placenta had remained in the womb. Nelly returned to the clinic to get instruments and intravenous injections, while Clemente attended the mother. Clemente realized the woman was bleeding to death, so he applied traditional techniques. When Nelly returned, they worked hard to save her, but she died that night. However, they agreed that they had effectively supported each other and done what they could to save the woman.

Members of some communities at first were unaccustomed to the presence of a CHW and devised ways of controlling the situation. A serious problem arose in the community of Pekereke with a CHW, Adolfo, when its members accused him of being a *kharisiri* (fat-snatcher). Doctors, nurses, and priests are frequently suspected of being *kharisiris*. Already discussed, kharisiris are legendary figures in Andean culture who steal people's fat. Andeans believe that fat provides energy and is as important as blood: to lose one's fat is to be stripped of energy and power. *Kharisiris* remove the fat with tubelike instruments. To call Adolfo a *kharisiri* is like calling a doctor a "bloodsucker."

Adolfo had been a mediocre CHW from the beginning. For two years, he had shown little enthusiasm and had infrequently attended the sick. When the people of Pekereke criticized him, he interpreted it as their rejection of him. They wanted another promoter. Elders avoided him and mothers didn't want him to examine their children and refused to assist at meetings of the mothers' club. They thought he was a *kharisiri* because he was giving so many injections, which they interpreted as "snatching fat." He had violated the rule that health promoters should only give injections when there is a written order from a doctor. Once he was labeled a *kharisiri*, his work as promoter stopped. To steal fat is contradictory to the role of Andean leadership, which is to circulate fat.

From this case, supervisors learned the importance of educating community members about their responsibility to collaborate with the promoter in public health measures. Subsequently, doctors and nurses began instructing members of the community several months before the election of a new health promoter. Members of the community elected a candidate after they and the supervisors negotiated on what the role of the health promoter was to be and how the promoter was to fit into the leadership structure of the community as well as the Ministry of Health. They were thus able to adapt health care to the complex and varied political structures of an Andean community.

The Adaptation: Making the Promoter Fit In

With the lesson of Pekereke in mind, project supervisors hoped to adapt the role of health promoter to existing political roles at the local or community level. However, political roles vary within Bolivian communities (see Abercrombie 1986; Albo 1985; Albo et al. 1989; Carter and Mamani 1989; Crandon-Malamud 1991; Handelman 1975; McEwen 1975; Rasnake 1988; and Smith 1989). Many Andean communities have *sindicatos* (peasant unions), which were instituted after the Bolivian Agrarian Reform (1954) (Bastien 1978:62–64, Buechler and Buechler 1971; Carter 1965). Community *sindicatos* are the base of a pyramidal organization topped by the Ministerio de Asuntos Campesinos. They are an important political feature of modern Bolivia. *Sindicatos* have overlapping, shifting fields of force from government officials to political parties and regional leaders and interests. Project Concern and the Ministry of Health wisely avoided placing the role of health promoter within the *sindicato* structure, because of its factionalism and politics associated with the MNR (Movimiento Nacionalista Revolucionario) (see Albo 1985:58–60; Albo et al. 1989:70–71).

Some communities maintain the traditional *cargo* system, such as discussed by Eric Wolf (1985), described for Kaata, Bolivia, by Bastien (1978:61–62), and analyzed in other Bolivian communities by Abercrombie (1986) and Rasnake (1988). Leadership is not something aspired to that benefits the individual; it is rather a specific burden *(cargo)* that needs to be assumed as one's responsibility to the community. The community embodies this leadership and shares it with individuals, who are expected to fulfill periodically the economic, labor, and time demands of it. *Cargos* vary, but some typical roles are those of *alcalde* (mayor), *alcalde escolar* (inspector of schools), *preste* (sponsor of fiesta), and *corregidor* (sheriff). Community members nominate men usually and women occasionally to these roles, but always in progression from the least to the most prestigious office. Peasants frequently resist nomination because of expenses involved in sponsoring rituals and feeding people during fiestas. With election comes prestige and the status of *pasado runa* (elder) and thus a leader within the community. In a sense, one becomes an adult in the Andean community by carrying the *cargos*. Although the graded

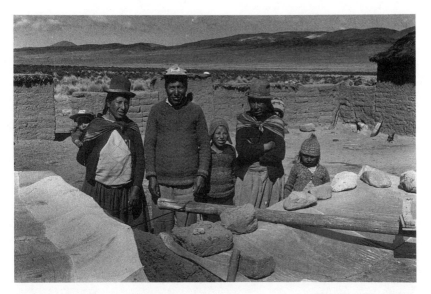

Male community health worker in the Department of Oruro, Altiplano, Bolivia, at 13,500 feet, teaching members of the community how to make a solar garden. They can grow tomatoes, cabbage, onions, and carrots in these gardens.

scale of *cargos* implies a hierarchy of prestige, it reflects the Andeans' appreciation for people who have served as guides in the community and their respect for elders as repositories of wisdom rather than as aspirants to control.

Cargo leadership does not accrue power and wealth to an individual, but rather prestige and a chance to grow up as a fully recognized "adult" in the community. An essential characteristic of *cargo* roles is that individuals receive their leadership "energy" from the community and then circulate it for the good of the community. By sponsoring rituals, leaders circulate community resources to feed all members and distribute symbolic foods (coca, llama fetuses and fat, and guinea pig blood) to the earth shrines so that Mother Earth feeds the community.

Symbols of leadership in the Andes are blood and fat. According to old Andean belief, blood is associated with life and comes from the heart, and fat is associated with energy and comes from the bowels. Leaders in Kaata, for example, are anointed on the heart and forehead with llama fat. In anointing and fertility rites, Kaatans rub the person and object with llama fat (Bastien 1978:54). Fat and blood, fluid and systemic symbols are external attributes of leaders, whose role is to circulate life and energy throughout the social and ecologi-

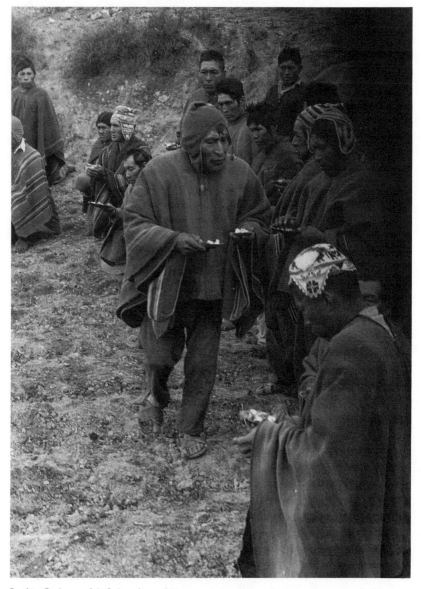

Sarito Quispe, chief ritualist of Kaata, giving llama fat to community leaders, a sign that they have been given the authority to be leaders. They will also feed llama fat to the earth shrines.

cal levels. By sponsoring rituals, leaders set in motion vital principles that unite the community into a social and metaphorical whole.

Supervisors Gregory Rake, Angela Lutena, and Oscar Velasco adapted the role of health promoter to *cargo, sindicato,* and *ayllu* leadership functions found in Bolivian communities. In accordance with *cargo* leadership, they envisioned the role of health promoter as a prestation of medical service to the community that is bestowed on a qualified member by the community for a limited period (three years) without a salary. Relative to *sindicato* leadership, supervisors requested that a secretary of health and members of a *comite de salud* (health committee) be elected from the same community as the promoter. The secretary of health and health committee were to collaborate with the promoter. Equally important, planners endeavored to incorporate the role of health promoter into the social and cultural structure of the *ayllu* in communities where it still functions as a principle of organization.

By combining *cargo* and *sindicato* leadership functions, supervisors avoided associating the role of promoter exclusively with a conservative or traditional view of Andean leadership. Scholars report that indigenous community leaders have resisted innovations and rejected officials from the state system (Inca, Spanish, Bolivian, or Ministry of Health) whose policies conflict with the principles of reciprocity and symbolic patterns that continue to define the *ayllu* (Earls 1973; Rasnake 1988). Ethnographic studies provide evidence that certain Andeans have world views that stress reciprocity and regulation rather than hierarchy and control (Schaedel 1988:772). Regulation implies that ordering is a systemic principle embodied more in the community and is the shared responsibility of all members rather than an individual principle entrusted to or found in someone. In the simplest human societies, regulation is shared by most or all of the adults in the community and ordering relies implicitly upon sacred propositions and sanctions (Adams 1981). Its cognitive patterns express little in the way of rigid hierarchization, whereas the regulatory and controlling mechanisms of a state society, which is explicitly based on an authority structure backed by coercive force, yield a cognitive pattern that legitimizes hierarchy.

Although these views provide keen insights into contemporaneous Andean communities—and, indeed, reciprocity and regulation through elaborate ritual systems are a key element of leadership—the problem for health planners is to incorporate these patterns of continuity into the emergent role of health promoter, who, as part of the community, must fit into its political dynamic and, as part of the dominant medical institution, must respond to its control.

The Community: A Shared Discourse Strategy

Culture is an engagement with the present mediated by the past. Andean communities are constituted not so much by shared values or common understanding, but rather by a "shared discourse in which alternative strategies, misunderstandings, conflicting goals and values are threshed out" (Smith 1989:234). Health promoters were asked to participate at rituals as a form of shared discourse where strategies of health are worked out for the sick person. Another form was the involvement of promoters with Andean institutions, such as *ayllu, minka* (reciprocal exchange of labor for goods), *mit'a* (labor service owed to the government by a male adult recognized as a member of the community), and *ayni* (reciprocal exchange of labor), so that they could negotiate with community members on how to use these strategies for public health.

A basic premise of primary health care is community participation, which translates for health planners as group dynamics or community development. This is a narrow view in that the basis for community participation is the way members of a community use certain cultural institutions as frameworks (rules of the game) for determining how they will adapt to the changing environment. Crucial for health workers is their knowing the rules of these institutions and, most important, how well they can play the game and win one for public health. Obviously an old-timer has an edge.

The *ayllu* is one expression of stability, flexibility, and strategy in Andean communities. Often elusive to scholars, it is described as a flexible Andean organizational form with its roots in the pre-Hispanic past. A pervasive characteristic of the *ayllu* and Andean community is reciprocity. The *ayllu* is also a discourse strategy involving land, lineage, community, cosmology, and economics in that it has many metaphorical, isomorphic, telluric, genealogical, political, and economic meanings. Ritual and divinations are frequently the arenas of these discourses, where people try to arrive at shared meanings for some objective (see Bastien 1978).

As an illustration: for changing political reforms, Kallawayas adapted *ayllu* Kaata and the traditional *cargo* system to land reform and the *sindicato* system. Traditionally, leaders of Kaata practiced a modified form of the *cargo* system and were called *jilacatas*. They carried out a variety of functions, such as overseeing the maintenance of paths, fences, and irrigation canals; handling bureaucratic and legal formalities demanded by the state; and leading the community through the ritual cycle. *Jilacatas* played major roles in sponsoring three major *ayllu* rituals, each dedicated to the selection of fields, first-plowing, and first-planting (see Bastien 1978:51–83). All Kaatans participated in these rituals and believed that if they fed coca and llama blood and fat to the earth shrines of Mount Kaata then Mother Earth *(Pachamama)* would provide them with a good harvest.

In 1954, agrarian reform laws ordered communities to form *sindicatos*, each with twelve secretary roles, such as secretary general, secretary of roads, secretary of sports, and secretary of animals. Kaatans adapted the legislated secretary roles into perduring Andean leadership roles (see Smith 1989). Although no longer called *jilacatas*, newly appointed secretaries have incorporated ritual activities characteristic of the *jilacatas*. When they ritually feed earth shrines on the three levels, the secretaries maintain the relationship between *ayllu* Kaata, its people, and agriculture. Leadership is transformed into complementary functions of not only coordinating people as secretaries according to the agrarian reform but also of sponsoring rituals that symbolically unite people, agriculture, land, and *ayllu*. Moreover, Kaatans continue to name secretaries according to the hierarchical ladder of the *cargo* system, even though they stage elections.

Ritual is an enacted discursive strategy par excellence in the Andes, and health workers must be skilled in it to be effective leaders. Isbell (1978), van den Berg (1990), and Zuidema (1964) have also shown the interrelationship of political and ritual roles. Within the Bolivian Andes, there is a close relationship among economic, political, social, ritual, and medicinal activities (Crankshaw 1980, 1983). Rituals function as discursive mechanisms of social organization, personal well-being, and the universe. The medical texts ethnomedical practitioners in the Andes refer to are the symbols of ritual, from divination with coca leaves to elaborate metaphorical meals for their ancestors and earth shrines. Discussed in chapter 4, the conflict between an auxiliary nurse and shaman in the village of Qaqachaka, Department of Oruro, was resolved only after the nurse participated in a curing ritual and began feeding the *ayllu* shrines (Bastien 1989, 1988a). Andeans perceive the causes of illnesses as a breach in the reciprocal relationship of themselves with their land, *ayllu*, and relatives, which must be redressed in ritual (Bastien 1978:129–49; van den Berg 1990). If health promoters aren't skilled ritual participants, they need to collaborate with ritualists who are. The lesson is that effective health leadership in the Andes must be a shared discourse that includes not only physical and biological intervention but also ritual regulation.

By 1984, three years after the promoter project began in Oruro, directors realized some of the above and accepted the following guidelines: the role of health promoters should be less one of hierarchy, control, and authority and more one of regulation, ritual activity, negotiation, and reciprocal services for health matters within the community. Doctors and nurses found this change difficult, and frequently reverted to being models of authoritarianism, discipline, and dogmatism. I conducted numerous workshops with doctors and nurses to correct this problem and had relative success in that several doctors changed their leadership roles. The duration of this success lasted only several years until Project Concern and the Ministry of Rural Health lost interest and reestablished the authoritarian/hierarchical structure that doctors and nurses were more comfortable with.

The Economics: Andean Resources and Institutions

Recompense of CHWs throughout the world is a major concern. As already mentioned, health promoters in Oruro were not paid a salary, but they could provide their skills in return for another service, which is an important Andean economic system referred to as *ayni* (exchange).

Aynisiña is a basic Aymara institution wherein peasants set up a system of prestation and counterprestation regarding work tasks. For example, someone helps another person thatch his roof. The recipient or his children now owe the helper an *ayni* for roof thatching or an equivalent task, due at some future time. Health promoters frequently use *ayni* in return for their work. A health promoter may donate a week at a training course or take care of a sick person for a week. In exchange, members of the community in the first instance and, in the second, the sick person, or his or her relatives, owe the health promoter an equivalency of work, such as herding the promoter's sheep or plowing a field. Health promoters used *ayni* during the drought (1982–1984) when they encouraged labor exchanges and cooperation in the community to prevent the hoarding of water as well as other conflicts. Promoters coordinated the activities of digging wells, routing water, and building irrigation canals. One creative way they used *ayni* was to have the family of the treated sick person do some public health service, such as build a latrine or dig a sewage ditch, in return for treatment by the health promoter. Another method of exchange is *turqasiña* (exchange), which refers to bartering produce for equitable produce. Health promoters utilize this practice when patients cannot pay for medicine but can provide some produce instead. The health promoters get the produce at a discount rate; they consume, exchange, or sell it at markets in Oruro, using the money to buy medicines. Payment in produce is a problem in Project Concern in Cochabamba because the rotating medical fund is maintained ultimately with convertible currency (U.S.$). CHWs who accept payment in kind cannot easily turn this into cash. However, they are supposed to replenish their stock of medicines using Bolivian pesos. Consequently, their stock is poorly maintained—a chronic problem (Timothy Wright, pers. com. 1992).

Health promoters also encouraged and assisted peasants in exchanging their local produce, such as potatoes, for that of another region, such as fruit or meat, thus balancing their diet. A nutritional problem for peasants exists in that they sell their produce to buy the consumer goods of industrialized society, such as Coca-Cola, cigarettes, canned goods, noodles, and drinking alcohol (190 proof).

Health promoters used *turqasiña* by during the years of hyperinflation in Bolivia. The hyperinflation began with the inordinate increase in public spending in 1982 (Cole 1987:39–64) and the cocaine trade. With a fragile tax system and ever-shrinking GDP, the effect was to set off the worst inflationary rate in the world since the last days of the Weimar Republic: 330 percent in 1983, 2,300 percent in 1984, and an annual rate of 29,800 percent in the first eight months of 1985. Health promoters advised peasants not to sell their produce for Bolivian pesos, which deflated at astronomical figures, but to store and exchange it for other produce. As protection against inflation, several health promoters taught their villagers to store surplus beets by a pre-Columbian method called *k'airo*, burying the beets beneath the earth and covering them with herbs.

When the government consequently ordered peasants to sell specified amounts of produce, health promoters took measures to increase productivity by introducing *huertas con carpas solares* (gardens with solar covers). These consisted of trenches approximately a meter deep, two meters wide, and three meters long, covered by clear plastic sheets. Intense solar radiation heated these gardens enough to prevent frost and freezing and to permit the cultivation of onions, carrots, tomatoes, beets, turnips, and radishes at altitudes above 4,000 m. In 1985, in the village of Sora Sora, Celestino, a health promoter introduced these hothouses, and within two years every family in the community was growing vegetables. This not only alleviated ailments caused by vitamin deficiencies but also initiated the marketing of surplus vegetables in Sora Sora during the *feria* on Wednesday, established for that purpose.

Since health promoters were unsalaried, they were little affected by the monetary devaluation or by subsequent stringent cutbacks in public spending beginning with the new economic policy of President Victor Paz, August 1985. Salaried medical personnel were repeatedly on strike to increase their wages; doctors went on strike thirteen times in 1983 and 1984. As best they could, health promoters provided a primary health delivery system for many peasants. The result was that health promoters depended more on Andean resources, ingenuity, and community support than on Project Concern, the Ministry of Health, and national economics. In 1988, 130 health promoters formed their own association independent of Project Concern and the Ministry of Health. They have elected officers and meet regularly to discuss ways to improve their skills in both ethno- and biomedicine. They realize that their grievances with doctors and nurses is better handled by group solidarity.

Hostility between health promoters and ethnomedical practitioners is a major obstacle in the collaborative health efforts of members of the community. In small Andean villages, many members are related either to ethnomedical practitioners or the health promoter, so that professional interests become lineage property, often resulting in feuds. Project Concern and the Ministry of Health encourage the selection of ethnomedical practitioners for training as health promoters as well as the continuation of ethnomedicine once they become health promoters. One-fourth of the health promoters in the Oruro project practice ethnomedicine as either midwives, herbalists, diviners, or shamans. I also conducted courses on ethnomedicine, Andean religion, and medicinal plants to help health promoters, as well as doctors and nurses, integrate biomedicine with ethnomedicine.

Olimpio Choque: Promoter and Curandero

Olimpio Choque is a renowned *curandero* who became a promoter. The son of Olimpio had been selected by the people of Calasaya, a community of 200 families, to be promoter, but died before the course began. Olimpio had suffered from *susto* (fright) and for a cure read the coca leaves, which said, "You are *asustado* (frightened)

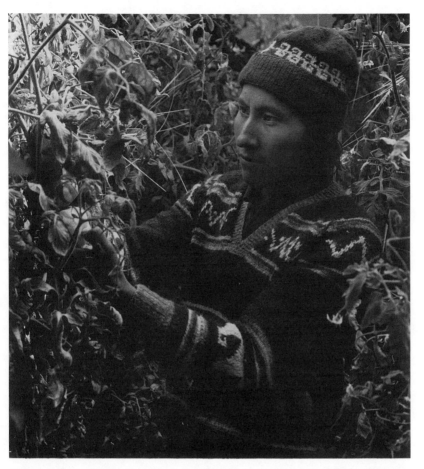

Community health worker Norberto Mamani, community of Qulta, Department of Oruro, built this solar garden to grow tomatoes. Other community
members followed his example, permitting them to supplement their carbohy-
drate diet of mostly potatoes.

because your son is calling you to take his place." Yet Olimpio worried that the role of health promoter would contradict his role as
ritualist and herbalist.

After his training, Olimpio returned to Calasaya, where he was
the elder of the health promoters in the Totora region. He diagnosed cases of leishmaniasis in his community. Popularly called *uta*
or *mal de los Andes*, mucocutaneous leishmaniasis is caused by a para-
site, carried by the sandfly, that eats away the nose cartilage and
disfigures the face (see Valdizán and Maldonado 1922, 1:288–91). Doctors and nurses infrequently see this disease because its victims fear

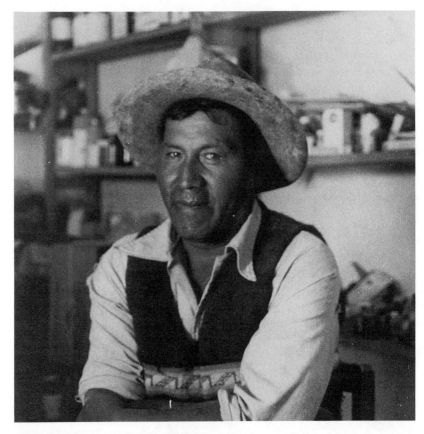

Olimpio Choque uses biomedicine and ethnomedicine in his *curandero* practice.

being seen by strangers and being placed in "leper colonies." Peasants often interpret this malady as punishment for breaking a taboo. Because Olimpio was a trusted *curandero*, he convinced the leishmaniasis patients to go to Oruro for treatment. Accompanying them, Olimpio asked Dr. Oscar Velasco, director of health promoters, for an authorization letter stating that after the patients were treated, they would be allowed to return to Calasaya. This set a precedent for inviting similar patients in other communities to seek treatment.

Olimpio also incorporated Andean religion into his practice as health promoter. On one occasion, he invited Dr. Velasco to worship at a *chullpa* (burial house) shrine for ancestors. Oscar accompanied him as they sprinkled alcohol to the east and west, where the sun rises and sets. Next, they sprinkled it on the ground for those sleeping in the earth, saying, "Don't forget us, help us in our work, and grant us health." They drank libations of alcohol, giving some to *Pachamama* (Mother Earth). From that moment, health promoters of Totora no longer considered Oscar as someone apart from them in his role as doctor and supervisor. As he described it, "When I left Calasaya they asked for my address and said, 'Now we are going to visit you and sleep in your house.' "

Later, Olimpio went to Oscar's home in Oruro to consult with him about his illness of *susto*. Trained in clinical psychiatry, Oscar did not undertake this type of therapy and introduced Olimpio to another *curandera*, Doña Matilda of Oruro. Matilda performed a ritual table *(mesa)* to feed the earth shrines, similar to that described for Kaata. The nightmares stopped and Olimpio regained confidence in himself and his work. Thus, Oscar and Matilda helped Olimpio resolve his grief over the death of his son as well as the conflict of his being a shaman who practiced biomedicine and ethnomedicine. Oscar did this by affirming the use of Andean rituals and practitioners in the therapy of Olimpio. Belief and participation in the rituals of native healers created an experience that spanned the differences of cultures, times, and histories and confirmed a policy that encourages health promoters to use Andean rituals for healing.

Olimpio had a *mallku* (shrine) within an Inca site, which he said provided him with the healing power of his ancestors. It was in the shape of a puma, a jaguar, whose symbolism is basic to Chavín, Tiahuanaco, and Cuzco, centers of Andean civilization. Olimpio led members of the community and promoters in a fiesta of *willancha* (blood sprinkling) to his *mallku*. They sacrificed a sheep, scattered its blood on the earth and *mallku*, and petitioned the earth for the health of the community.

Health promoters who followed Olimpio's ideas of incorporating Andean religion into their medical practices called it *Religión Andina* and said it was a form of living and of being in communion with each other and with nature. They believed in the history of their ancestors not as a return to the past but rather as a revitalization of the present with a meaningful tangential connection through ritual. Setha Low (1988) observed that as the technological "magic" of medical practice challenges religious healing's claim to miraculous power, the number of lay, quasi-religious cults increases, sacralizing medical symbols by placing them within religious contexts. The health promoters of Oruro were encouraged to embed Western technological medicine within the symbolic context of Andean culture.

Of the 130 promoters in the Department of Oruro, the majority are active health workers, well accepted and supported by members of their communities. They have effected many changes: latrines, gardens, reforestation, and new agricultural products. They have been active in immunization campaigns. They have coordinated efforts between bio- and ethnomedical practitioners. The promoter project in Oruro has been used as a model for similar programs in Cochabamba, Potosí, Sucre, and Tarija in Bolivia. It is considered a key to the success of primary health care in Bolivia.

Conclusions

Successful health workers have been those who are actively involved with members of the community for innovating health changes. The most successful are those who share and practice the beliefs and customs of the people of the community. With regard to culture, they have the same values and traditions as the peasants of their community; but with regard to health, they are innovators of bio-medicine. They are sensitive, however, to the integration of biomedi-cine and ethnomedicine. Part of the success of health promoters in Oruro is that they adapt to Aymara and Quechua styles of leader-ship, which are embedded in the cultural, social, ritual, and cosmo-logical system of the *ayllu* and community. Part of health promoter training should include the recognition and encouragement of this embedment through the use of Andean rituals, symbols, and folk-lore. This would encourage the candidate to become immersed in the cultural context.

As Andean people adapt biomedicine to their culture, health promoters can assist in this process. It is necessary, however, that planners and directors of health promoter projects understand ways that the roles, beliefs, and practices of biomedicine can articulate with indigenous roles, ethnomedicine, political structures, and eco-nomics. Because the latter roles and structures vary greatly between cultures and between communities within the same culture, health promoters can serve as negotiators in the type of primary health care that the community needs and will accept.

6

Midwives and Maternal and Infant Health Care

WITH NANCY EDENS

The majority of babies born (60–80 percent) in the developing world are delivered by midwives and traditional birth attendants (TBAs) where there are no alternative midwifery services in rural communities (Isenalumbe 1990). Midwives are men and women who are involved with the entire pregnancy and delivery process, and TBAs are those who only assist the mother at the time of birth. Although some practices of midwives and TBAs need to be modified to ensure the safe care of the mother and child, there is even greater need for doctors and nurses to treat the midwives and TBAs with respect and begin to incorporate them into the health-care system. The integration of midwives and TBAs into public health programs is necessary to improve maternal and child health worldwide.

An effective way to integrate TBAs and midwives into primary health care is through domiciliary midwifery services. Pregnancy and childbirth are normal physiological processes, which for healthy women can almost always be successfully completed with minimal assistance and less stress in the home. A study of domiciliary midwifery services in a suburban area of Benin City, Nigeria, indicated that mothers liked TBAs and midwives mainly because they delivered babies in the home (Isenalumbe 1990). In Benin, hospitals were congested, so a pilot project was set up in 1976 to take simple midwifery skills to women in their homes. When an expectant mother visits the clinic for the first time, her obstetric and gynecological history is obtained. Those considered at risk are referred to the hospital for antenatal care and delivery. Risk factors are primiparity (age less than eighteen years), grand multiparity (five or more pregnancies), age over thirty-five years, adverse obstetric history, and pregnancy less than twelve months after the last delivery. Mothers not at risk are encouraged to deliver at home and are visited by a midwife to assess the suitability of the home environment, such as the availability of a well-lighted area. When labor begins, mothers

137

ask for assistance from one of the midwives on call (Isenalumbe 1990).

Domiciliary midwifery services have been satisfactorily received by mothers in Benin. Not only for Benin but also for other communities as well, these services provide a means of integrating midwives into primary health care and improving maternal and child health.

The first task for those working toward integration is to conduct research that evaluates the practices and competencies of midwives and TBAs. The array of services and levels of expertise offered by midwives and TBAs are as varied as the cultures in which they practice their craft (see Kay 1982). They may be male or female; a relative of the mother or a full-time practitioner; a ritualist who directs the mother before, during, and after birth; or someone who only delivers the baby. Programs that endeavor to include midwives and TBAs into the national health policy need to adjust the training and expected changes to fit the cultural practices and values of these practitioners and their patients. Positive or neutral practices should be encouraged for the emotional and cultural support they provide the mother and her family. Unhealthy practices can only be changed after establishing a trusting and respectful relationship between the doctors and nurses and the midwives and TBAs. Establishing this type of relationship will be easier when the positive and neutral traditional activities are allowed to remain in practice. This is because the practitioners and clients will feel more respected and in control of their lives in spite of the changes that are taking place.

Childbirth in Bolivia

Most doctors and nurses assume that only they should deliver babies, in the particular way they were trained, and in a clinic or hospital. The following case from Bolivia provides an example of doctors trying to change traditional practices of midwives without an adequate understanding of that tradition (Bastien 1987:77–78).

In 1981, doctors in Oruro, Bolivia, advocated that midwives have expectant mothers lie down during delivery instead of squatting, as is customary throughout the region. Doctors feared that the newborn would emerge too rapidly and injure its head on the concrete floor. Not one of them had ever seen a midwife deliver a baby, so Oscar Velasco, director of traditional medicine, invited them to one such birth. The midwife gave the mother a tea made from anise, a commonly used oxytocic, when she was at the height of labor. The

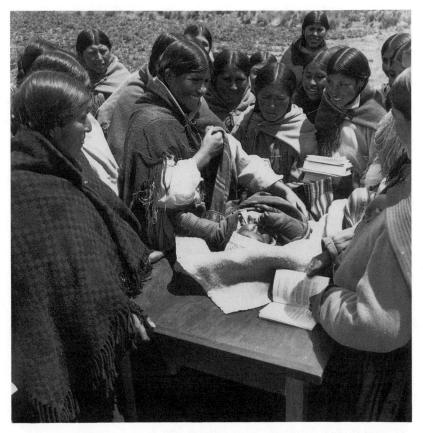

Aymara midwife instructing traditional birth assistants and midwives in Challapata, Department of Oruro.

mother squatted over a thick sheepskin rug, close to the earthen floor, and as the baby arrived, the midwife received the head in her palms. The umbilical cord was cut with scissors—short for girls and long for boys (symbolic of the penis). The infant's eyes were shielded to protect them from any bright light. To ensure this protection, the birthing room was kept dark except for candles. After the delivery, the husband brought his exhausted wife a bowl of sheep soup to give her strength.

After observing the birth, the doctors discussed with the midwife details that should be changed and those that should be left alone. They conceded that squatting is better than the supine position. There is scientific evidence supporting this (Haire 1972:21–22; Howard 1951, 1958; Mengert and Murphy 1933), which is fortunate since getting women to change the birth position is as difficult as changing dietary habits. The emphasis of the discussion was to change only those aspects that were prejudicial or dangerous to the health of the mother and child. With the motto, "Go with the Andean system and improve it," doctors began to think as midwives would and to devise ways of improving traditional delivery practices.

For instance, the doctors noticed that the sheepskin rug was dirty, so at the meetings of the *Clubes de Madres* (or Mothers' Clubs, the association found in 3,000 Bolivian communities), the doctors suggested that an expectant mother be instructed to wash the sheepskin in soap and water and dry it in the sun. This is an excellent antiseptic procedure that can be done easily by the midwife or mother before delivery.

The doctors also learned that the mother often drinks oxytocic teas and coffee very early in the labor, causing her to be too exhausted for the delivery. Because the vegetal oxytocics are not as controllable or powerful as synthetic drugs, midwives and mothers need to know when an oxytocic is needed and exactly when to administer it, namely at the moment when the mother feels like she has to go to the toilet (in terms that she understands) or when she is in danger of hemorrhaging.

Misuse of oxytocics might not be uncommon. Midwives in Haiti place onions and peppers into the vagina of a pregnant woman with a prolonged delivery to draw the baby out. The onions and peppers may swell the tissues and muscles, making the delivery more painful and difficult to manage (Gretchen Berggren, pers. com. 1990). Doctors and nurses could advise in such cases.

By attending traditional births, Bolivian doctors learned a lot about their patients: that the bright lights and white-colored walls of their delivery rooms were unpopular among Andean mothers, that doctors should not refuse to allow the family to bring sheep soup into the clinic for the mother after delivery (the family usually smuggles it in anyway), and that it is extremely important they not cut a boy's umbilical cord too short (to Bolivians, this would inhibit the normal development of the penis). These insights led to possible explanations for why many Andeans refused to have their babies delivered in clinics and hospitals.

These doctors were not advocating the use of clinics for all deliveries (an estimated 95 percent of the babies born in Bolivia are normal deliveries attended by midwives and TBAs). Their intent was to instruct the midwives on how to recognize complicated pregnancies, refering these cases to them. For new clinics, it was decided to decrease the lights in the delivery room, paint the walls in dark colors, and abolish the rule against bringing in food to patients.

Understandably, the doctors were concerned about germs, so they suggested that midwives wash their hands, use sterilized gloves, and cut the umbilical cord with a disinfected razor blade. The gloves were seldom used because the midwive's hands were coarse and calloused, having little dexterity as it was, and the gloves diminished it. Moreover, the gloves were saved for butchering animals. Although the doctors suggested that a new razor blade be used for each birth, the midwives saw this as too wasteful and insisted on recycling the blade. Thus, the doctors taught the midwives to sterilize the blade with fire and alcohol.

At times, biomedical technicians advocate measures, such as the use of disposable syringes and razor blades, that are important to curtail contagious diseases but not adopted because peasants are thrifty, ecologically oriented, and unaware of how diseases spread. Peasants infrequently throw syringes and razor blades away, but when they do, someone else salvages them.

There is an ecological issue involved in persuading people in developing nations to throw some things away. Not only is the peasant's access to resources limited but also the cost of disposables is prohibitive. Whenever possible, biomedical technology needs to be responsive to the needs and resources of the population. Peasants can be taught to use medically safe techniques that conserve their limited resources. For example, instead of using disposables, they can boil the syringe between each use or sterilize the razor blade by holding it over a match and cleaning it with alcohol. Rather than using rubber gloves, midwives can be taught to properly wash their hands and clean their fingernails before a delivery. Another major problem with the gloves, if they are utilized for a birth, is that midwives do not dispose of them after the delivery. They use them for numerous deliveries as well as for butchering meat and cleaning up dirty substances. In their minds, the gloves are to protect the hands, not to prevent the spread of bacteria.

In subsequent meetings, the midwives were instructed in ways to refine their practice that would meet standards acceptable to both them and the doctors. The midwives were then presented with midwife kits provided by UNICEF, that were packaged in shiny aluminum cases. After a year, the aluminum cases were replaced with cloth backpacks because the Indians feared that the shiny metallic cases attracted *thunupa* (lightning), a dreaded deity with a lethal charge, especially on the Altiplano, where annually a dozen or so people are killed by it. The doctors then realized that the shiny aluminum and steel equipment in their clinics and hospitals probably had a similar effect on the peasants—revealing possibly another reason why there is such a low utilization of modern medical facilities by Andeans. By observing the midwives and having discussions with them, the doctors learned, firsthand, the importance of following traditional practices and that both ethno- and biomedicine benefit from a doctor-midwife communication and exchange of information.

Variations of Midwifery throughout the World

Guatemalan Midwives. In many regions of Guatemala midwives are elderly widows with no other source of income and who get little respect for their work. An exception are the midwives who practice around Lake Atitlan in the Guatemalan Highlands (Paul 1975; Paul and Paul 1975). They are ritualists who attend to the mother pre- and postpartum as well as during the birth. Marked at birth by the presence of a caul (when part of the amniotic sack covers the baby's head), which foretells their role as birth assistants, they are further called to be midwives by dreams, visions, and omens as they grow older.

Because the peasants of Lake Atitlan perceive pregnancy as an imbalance, it is the role of the midwife to help the mother regain homeostasis in physical, emotional, and social dimensions. In addition, the midwife may foretell the baby's future and perform prophylactic rituals if negative signs appear, such as a looped umbilical cord. A week after delivery, the midwife performs another ritual to demarcate the end of the imbalance and to reintegrate the mother into the community. Midwives and their rituals assure safe deliveries to prospective mothers when they feel especially vulnerable. Moreover, the roles of the midwife, other than assistance at the time of delivery, are especially important to the peasants of Lake Atitlan because of their perception of pregnancy as a time of physical and social imbalance.

Malaysian Midwives. Malaysian midwives are highly respected and competent women who deal with physical and spiritual aspects of pregnancy and motherhood (Karim 1984). They inherit the role of midwife through their matrilineage and further learn about it through dreams. Learning through dreams earns greater respect as a form of acquiring knowledge than does the formal training the government midwives receive.

Malaysian midwives develop a motherlike relationship with their patients. With this bonding, midwives assume responsibility for a safe delivery and for maintaining family harmony. They possess supernatural powers to protect pregnant women from deities who inflict psychic, physical, and sometimes fatal injuries. They also treat the mother throughout pregnancy and after childbirth, being involved with not only pregnancy and delivery but also child care, nursing, weaning, and family planning—everything from menstrual disorders to abortions.

In comparison, Bolivian TBAs interviewed in 1987 in Cocapata, Department of Cochabamba, completely disassociate themselves from the responsibility of treating the child after birth. The infant mortality rate for this region is estimated around 140 per 1,000 live births, so if these TBAs were to get involved in neonatal care, they would be facing a high rate of mortality. When they were told that babies sometimes die from neonatal tetanus soon after birth (at about seven days) and that this is caused by contamination of the umbilical cord during delivery, they claimed that all the babies they delivered lived. They indicated that their role was to deliver babies alive, and if they got sick, it was the *curanderos'* responsibility to cure them.

Ghanaian Traditional Birth Attendants. In Ghana, West Africa, the typical TBA is approximately sixty-two years old. Two-thirds of the Ghanaian TBAs are farmers and 94 percent are illiterate. Slightly half of the TBAs are men, and of these, 79 percent are herbalists, whereas only 11 percent of the women TBAs are herbalists. The TBAs learn their skills from their parents and grandparents, and they practice part time. Male TBAs deliver an average of 8.5 babies a year and female TBAs, 4.4 babies a year. Although TBAs with herbal knowledge sometimes provide prenatal care with dietary advice, they usually only see the mother after labor begins, which provides no opportunity for prenatal detection of potential problems. TBAs pray over the mother for a safe delivery as their only form of ritual activity. Nevertheless, herbalist TBAs believe that some members of the community suspect them of using evil charms to harm the fetus. About 17 percent of Ghanaian women deliver their own babies and receive no formal instructions, learning only from experience (Ampofo et al. 1977:197–203; Neumann et al. 1974; Nicholas et al. 1976).

These cross-cultural examples suggest the variety of practices and responsibilities of midwives and TBAs found throughout the world. Because there is such cultural variance worldwide, integrated health training for midwives and TBAs should build upon their already existing expertise, practices, and sociocultural acceptability. Their training must incorporate the beliefs, practices, needs, and expectations specific to the people in each culture and community. If trainers accommodate cultural needs by encouraging positive and neutral practices to continue, the desired changes in negative practices will occur with less resistance. Often, innovative health practices are not perceived by the population as an improvement, so they are not adopted. An example is teaching sterile techniques to people who have no concept of germs. When changes in traditional techniques are adopted, it may be because the practitioners and patients have been treated with respect and been allowed to feel in control of their lives. Thus, they feel more comfortable with the changes in their lives (Jordan 1978:87).

Inappropriate Training for Midwives

Midwives and TBAs have frequently developed practices that are uniquely adapted to their competence, environment, resources, and clients. Because trainers often either discount the value of ethnomedicine or are uninformed about it, there are numerous instances when trainers have replaced healthy ethnomedical practices with unhealthy ones.

Cutting the Umbilical Cord. In Mexico, for example, health educators taught Maya midwives to cut the umbilical cord with scissors and then pack it with cotton balls soaked in alcohol (Jordan 1978:59, 84). This may have led to the increased rate of umbilical infection and neonatal tetanus because the scissors were more difficult to sterilize adequately and were used for other purposes and the stump was left moist. Traditionally, the midwives had cut the cord with a freshly cut bamboo splinter, cauterizing the stump with a candle flame and then dressing it with a burnt cloth. Using scissors was an inappropriate technology that had replaced an appropriate one (Gonzales and Behar 1966:86; Cosminsky 1974:286).

The same educators taught Maya midwives to cut the umbilical cord immediately after birth, which frequently deprived infants of up to 25 percent of their blood supply (Cosminsky 1974:287; 1977:85). This practice was promoted earlier by American obstetricians who were used to working in a hospital setting, although early cutting delays expulsion of the placenta and increases the possibility of maternal hemorrhage through retention of the placenta or its fragments (Haire 1972:25–26).

Another obstetric practice proven unhealthy because it places stress on the infant's heart is that of stripping or milking the umbilical cord by squeezing the cord blood toward the infant's naval (Haire 1972:25).

Herbal Teas. Health educators frequently discredit the efficacy of herbal medicines for pregnant mothers, and they teach midwives and TBAs to administer synthetic drugs. Synthetic drugs are easier to control, but they are also costly, sporadically available, and may have unknown effects on the mother and fetus (Cosminsky 1974:285–86; 1978:118–19; Haire 1972:19–20). Health educators often attempt to restrict the administration of any drug altogether. As mentioned earlier, many medicinal plants are effective oxytocics that cause contractions (Bastien 1978:78–79), and their use may be necessary to save a woman's life when she is in danger of hemorrhaging from a retained placenta. A large part of the indigenous midwife's particular expertise lies in an intimate and extensive knowledge of the use of local herbal resources (Cosminsky 1976:239). Many folklore remedies relieve nausea, pain, and the discomfort from milk retention as well as serve to reassure the mother ritually and symbolically.

Repositioning the Fetus. Sometimes health trainers dissuade midwives from massaging mothers for fear of improper handling. Midwives massage mothers to establish a closeness and to reassure them, to help them relax and prepare for the birth, to determine the position of the baby and, if necessary, to change it in order to prevent a breech presentation or a cesarean section (Cosminsky 1974:285–86, 1977:96; Greenburg 1982:1601; Jordan 1978:19–22). Maternal massage is the most widespread and popular traditional service rendered by midwives.

In Bolivia and other parts of Latin America, the Spanish introduced the sometimes dangerous use of the *manteo* (blanket) to reposition the baby. To use the *manteo*, four strong men hold the corners of a blanket on which the mother is suspended. While the midwife directs their movements, they reposition the baby by rolling and bouncing the mother. It is usually a gentle procedure, but there are reported cases when the mother was thrown into the air trampoline style to reposition the baby forceably. An even more dangerous, but infrequent, Bolivian practice is the insertion of the hand through the vagina and into the uterus to reposition the baby for delivery. With good reasons, health educators discourage midwives from employing either of these practices and encourage them to refer these cases to doctors.

Delivery Position. Another inappropriate method imposed on many women and midwives is delivery in the supine position, in which the mother lies on her back with her thighs flexed on her abdomen. Delivering a baby in this position instead of in the traditional squatting, kneeling, or sitting positions provides better visual access to the birth canal for the midwife, TBA, or doctor. However, the increased maternal pain and dangers to both the mother and infant's health renders this exportation of American obstetrical techniques wholly inappropriate during a rural home birth (Cosminsky 1977:95).

The supine position has many negative effects (Haire 1972; Howard 1951, 1958). It can adversely affect the mother's blood pressure, cardiac return, and pulmonary ventilation. It further inhibits the mother's voluntary efforts to push her baby out spontaneously, decreases the normal intensity of contractions, and causes the baby's supply of blood and oxygen to decrease. With the woman in this position, deliverers need to rely more on using forceps to increase the traction necessary for the delivery. It also inhibits the spontaneous expulsion of the placenta, significantly increasing the incidence of hemorrhaging. Because the supine position increases tension on the pelvic floor and stretches the perineal tissue, deliverers have to perform an episiotomy (incision of the perineum at the end of the second stage of labor to avoid laceration of the perineum and to facilitate delivery).

The practice of imposing a position that increases maternal and fetal distress—and in a technologically oriented setting, capable of handling complications in an aseptic manner—is questionable at best. But to teach the supine position to midwives who practice in isolated, nonsterile environments is medically unethical. As Sheila Cosminsky (1977:95) observed, the supine position reflects the value placed on efficiency and convenience for the obstetrician and on chemical interference of labor (see Jordan 1975). In a rural household, the supine position causes a more difficult, dangerous, and anxiety-provoking birth. Furthermore, exposure of female genitalia may be so contrary to the cultural norms for the treatment of women and the rules of modesty that this in itself can be considered harmful (Cosminsky 1977:82; Jordan 1978:83). For these reasons, it is not surprising that midwives and mothers have so vehemently resisted the use of the supine delivery position.

Evaluating the Technology. Because the innovations described above are still being promoted in many midwife training programs (Greenburg 1982), doctors and nurses need to evaluate whether an innovation is appropriate to the situation and environment the midwife or TBA is working in and whether it will cause a degree of improvement in care sufficient to justify the effort required to institute it. So many unhealthy practices need to be changed that it is counterproductive to concentrate on those practices which are insignificant or uniquely adaptive to a particular environment or culture and thus new to biomedically oriented trainers.

A number of questions can prompt answers for evaluating whether a biomedical practice is appropriate or inappropriate for midwives and TBAs to follow in any culture.

1. Is the change worth the effort? Some items are incidental, such as herbal teas, amulets, rituals, and dietary restrictions.

2. Does the change replace some practice that is more socially and economically feasible? Doctors have recommended that women give birth in clinics, but this is expensive and too impersonal for many mothers who want their babies delivered at home with the family present.

3. Given the environment, will the change improve or worsen conditions for the mother and child? For example, midwives from the Kallawaya of Curva encourage the mother to remain in bed a week after birth to avoid *wayra* (wind). Doctors maintain that this is wrong and that the mother should be up and around after giving birth. This may be maladaptive, however, in a region where strong winds frequently weaken debilitated mothers. Doctors also suggest that midwives wash the baby after birth, a practice midwives hesitate to do because they claim that the natural fluids protect the baby.

4. If midwives accept an innovation, how will this change their practice? How will the community accept this innovation? In Oruro, some midwives lost clientele once they had accepted elements of biomedicine. This points to the need to prepare the community for changes instituted by the midwife.

The answers to these questions should help determine how appropriate and well received an intended innovation will be for the midwives, TBAs, and their patients.

Customs and Cultural Norms

Further concerns in working with midwives are the influences of customs and cultural norms on their practices. In many instances, the objectives of health programs conflict with cultural patterns, such as religious ritual, deference to certain community members, and political organization (Foster 1958; Heggenhougen 1984; Paul and Demarest 1984). These patterns and rules must be considered for the desired changes to be successful.

An evaluation of a program for training midwives in Papua New Guinea revealed an intense fear of contact with uterine blood, which was believed to cause shortness of breath and weakness in not only the midwife but also her family. In response, the midwives requested that they be supplied rubber gloves (Schumacher 1987).

In Malaysia, conflicts arose between the traditional midwives, whose skills were inherited and revealed through dreams and visions, and the new government-trained midwives (Karim 1984). When the younger government midwives tried to supervise the older traditional midwives, the deference culturally expected by elders was disregarded. The conflicts resulted in accusations of witchcraft against the government midwives, which ensured that no one would utilize their services. The communities supported the traditional midwives rather than the government-trained midwives, who were young, unmarried, childless, and thus "inexperienced" and unqualified to deal with childbirth. Also, because the government-trained midwives had not acquired their skills through supernatural revelation, they could not offer the added service of providing supernatural protection for the mothers and their families.

That these types of conflicts occur should not be surprising. Cross-culturally, the majority of midwives and TBAs are older women who have survived childbearing years successfully, and are past the "dangerous" menstruating phase of life. The potential for conflicts between trained and untrained midwives needs to be studied before deciding who will be selected for training. Also, it is highly recommended that members of the community participate in making these decisions.

Acceptance or Rejection? Culturally determined procedures, such as proper disposal of the placenta and umbilical cord and cutting the cord to the culturally mandated length, should not only be allowed to continue at home births but also be accommodated in hospitals and clinics (I. Kelly 1955). Ceremonies and rituals should be encouraged for the assurance, comfort, and bonding with family and community that they provide the mother and child.

A careful assessment should be made of how certain customs and practices function within the cultural context for the mother, her family, and her community before any attempt is made to change them. If any cultural practice endangers the mother and child, then these practices must be replaced by healthy ones. For example, midwives in Cochabamba, Bolivia, used dust from the corners of the door to powder the freshly severed umbilical cord. This dust may harbor the tetanus spore, so it was recommended that they use fresh ashes, perhaps from burnt incense, instead. This compromise satisfied both medical and religious needs.

Food Habits. An area of maladaptive behavior often encountered is various eating habits and customs that do not provide the expectant and lactating mother with necessary proteins, vitamins, and minerals. Nutritional problems present the greatest danger to maternal and child health in the developing world (Fathalla et al. 1986; Sai et al. 1986), so eating restrictions that place a malnutritional burden on mothers and their children need to be modified. Also, malnutrition can delay the age of menarche and reduce fertility by suppressing ovulation, causing tragic results for those couples desiring children. Next to birthing customs, eating customs are among the most difficult to change because of the economic (access to nutritional resources), historical, religious, and symbolic purposes they fulfill within the society. Dietary practices originate in a variety of beliefs ranging from a need to maintain hot/cold, wet/dry balances within the body to observances of supernatural sanctions. They may be culturally mandated or idiosyncratic, voluntary or strictly enforced by the family and community (see Billington et al. 1963; Cosminsky 1977; Imperato 1977:131; Jenkins and Heywood 1984:11; Greenburg 1982:1600–1601; McElroy and Townsend 1985:222–64). Hence, dealing with eating customs requires an understanding of how these customs fit into the underlying cognitive perceptions of the people (see Jerome et al. 1980). Not all eating customs are detrimental. For example, midwives from many cultures prohibit the intake of salt and prescribe chicken or mutton soup after delivery. Unfortunately, all too often, food restrictions and customs disallow protein-rich foods, such as meat, eggs, and milk, or vitamin-rich fruits and vegetables at times when the mother and child need them the most.

Several studies have presented ways in which health educators can evaluate and mitigate detrimental food-related practices.

Jenkins and Heywood (1984:11,15) write that any attempts to change dietary behavior must be founded on a clear understanding of how dietary beliefs affect the maintenance of social structure and identity. They provide examples of how to elicit this information from local individuals. Cosminsky (1977:79) describes how, in Guatemala, perceptions of the hot/cold theory of a balanced diet can be incorporated into the medical system by the addition of certain hot or cold substances (chili or cinnamon) to neutralize the effects of an otherwise avoided food. I. Kelly (1955) suggests rehydrating infants in Mexico with traditional herbal teas since they are made from boiled and sterile water. Herbal teas in the Andes contain ample sugar and potassium, which provide a nearly complete rehydration formula, and salt often occurs in the water naturally. Kelly (1955) recommends stressing an especially healthy food source to compensate for missing elements rather than struggling to convince people to eat the restricted foods. Jordan (1978:30) and Cosminsky (1977:79) cite cases of midwives who successfully combined nutritional training with local food customs. Finnerman (1989:169) reports a similar mixing of local hot/cold humeral concepts with the use of pharmaceuticals.

A frequently encountered custom that should be discouraged is denying the newborn its mother's postpartum colostrum (a clear secretion that is present in the breasts before milk is produced) (Cosminsky 1977:89; Pratinidhi et al. 1985:116). The colostrum is especially rich in nutrients and antibodies that benefit the infant until its immune system has had a chance to develop. Also, midwives should be trained to encourage prompt breast-feeding because nipple stimulation causes uterine contractions that aid in the expulsion of the placenta, and thus reduces the risk of postpartum hemorrhage and the need for oxytocics. Breast-feeding also promotes early bonding between mother and child.

In the Altiplano of Bolivia, mothers wean their babies between the ages of one and two and feed them small portions of foods prepared for the family. Mothers give them small samplings so as to avoid *anteojo* (jealous stares) from the rest of the family. It is believed that *anteojo* causes diarrhea and *susto*. Altiplano children lose weight after weaning, and up to the age of five weigh considerably less than other children at similar ages (Oscar Velasco, pers. com. 1990).

Before 1950, Altiplano mothers prepared more nutritious and digestible foods for weaned children, foods that were rich in carbohydrates—especially necessary for children from ages one to two—such as gruel made from potato flour; chicha made from tender corn with little fermentation; *api*, a cereal drink from purple corn,

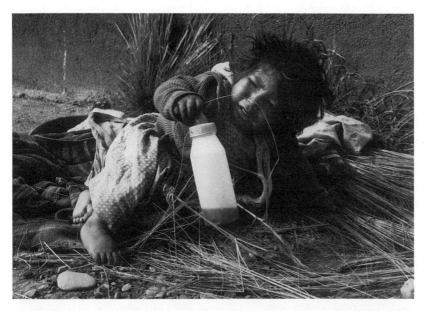

Bottle-feeding has been promoted by U.S. corporations making formulas. Infant mortality rates have increased in Bolivia because of unsterile methods in preparing the formula.

cinnamon, and sugar; and a drink prepared from sheep's milk and *willkaparu* corn. For coarser food, mothers masticated it first and gave it mouth to mouth to their children (Oscar Velasco, pers. com. 1990).

Even more detrimental to nutrition in Bolivia, a few ill-directed programs, mass media, and corporations introduced bottle-feeding, which increased morbidity and mortality, and placed economic hardships on families. Mothers abandoned breast-feeding so they could leave infants with younger children in order to work. They later realized that bottle feeding is a maladaptive innovation because unsterile water is used to dilute the formula and wash the bottles and nipples. Even if the importance of proper sterilization could be adequately conveyed to mothers in rural settings, the cost in fuel and time invested is prohibitive. Bottle-feeding results in decreased opportunity for mother/infant bonding, denies the infant's acquiring the mother's antibodies, and places an exorbitant burden on the family due to the cost of an unnatural commodity when a better, natural one is readily available.

In Bolivia and elsewhere, breast-feeding can aid in spacing births by suppressing ovulation so that lactating mothers become pregnant

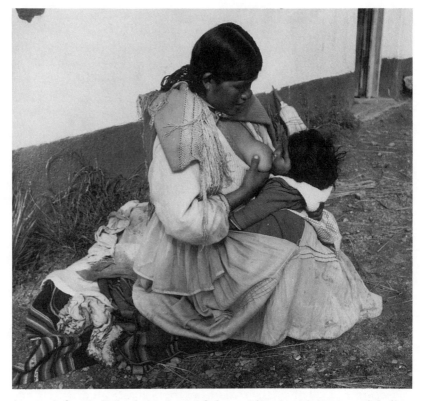

Aymara infant in Peñas being breast-fed, providing it with immunoglobulins, important in building resistance to disease and providing vital nutrients.

on an average of thirty-two months after the birth of a child, compared to eighteen months for nonlactating mothers. In spite of these well-known adverse effects of bottle-feeding (Dobbing 1988; Dobrin 1977; Margoulies 1977; Raphael 1980), working mothers continue to bottle-feed for convenience and out of perceptions of being "modern," as advertised. When the infant lacks certain nutrients, these should be supplemented in sterilized water and bottles, but in many cases, supplements are diluted beyond a nutritional advantage and with unsterile water by mothers trying to stretch the expensive commodity (Raphael 1976).

Many of the customs cited above conflict with what health promoters teach. These areas of potential conflict must be addressed and dealt with in the planning stage of a program, not after the damage has been done. The customs associated with pregnancy, delivery, and child care are especially numerous because these are times of great concern and danger, and they may vary tremendously from culture to culture. It is important that midwives and TBAs be encouraged to continue the customs and rituals unique to their clientele.

Traditional peoples often perceive of childbirth in mythological and cosmological dimensions. For example, Andeans interrelate the fertility and childbearing capacities of a woman to those of *Pachamama* (Mother Earth). Very traditional Quechuas still maintain that the man carries the male seed and the woman carries the female seed. Kallawayas told me that the sex of the child was determined by who reached orgasm first during intercourse. After a Kallawaya child is born, it is immediately given an earth shrine on the mountain and the placenta is buried in the patio of the house. Among other Andeans the placenta is kept, dried, and used as medicine.

Rituals. Birth for many peoples is a rite of passage that involves phases of separation, liminality, and incorporation (see Van Gennep 1960). Midwives and TBAs function as intermediaries who guide the mother and infant through these phases. They separate the mother from culturally perceived dangers—spirits, taboo places, and perhaps her husband—and protect her from a vast array of cosmological forces—baby snatchers, the dead, and other malevolent anthropomorphic and zoomorphic figures surrounding the community. For example, Quechuas of the Cochabamba Valley in Bolivia believe that neonatal tetanus is caused by witchcraft inflicted upon the mother, whom midwives can protect by performing rituals.

Midwives also separate the baby from the mother when they sever the umbilical cord, which has symbolic meanings in that one person is becoming two. For many people in traditional cultures, fertility and cosmogenic symbolism is embedded in the sacred. Midwives act as ritualists during the liminal phase of the instant after birth, when the infant has not yet breathed but is separated from the mother. This brief period is one of suspension, and the midwife is expected to assist the child take its first breath. The midwife introduces the infant to the air of the world. For the Quechua, this is *samay,* the vital circulating fluid that they breathe and which unites them with others. In the final phase of this ritual, the midwife reunites the baby with the mother and incorporates it into the family and the community. This part usually involves a meal: sheep soup for the mother, maternal milk for the infant, and produce from the father's land for the midwife.

Childbirth rituals demonstrate people's perceptions of their universe. This can be illustrated by Hopi and Cheyenne birth rituals. When a Hopi baby is born, the father's closest female relative, usually his mother or one of his sisters, arrives and washes the baby's head (Coolidge 1975:62–63). Four marks or lines of cornmeal are then placed on the four walls of the room. Every five days she again washes the baby's head, and each time one of the marks of cornmeal is removed from the wall. At the end of the twenty days, when the last mark is removed, she bathes the baby and puts cornmeal on its lips. She utters a prayer while strewing cornmeal toward the sun and in this prayer gives the baby its name.

The symbolism of four relates to the four directions of the Hopi universe. The father's female relative represents the importance of the Hopi's matrilineal society. Cornmeal symbolizes corn as their main food staple; the sun is important for growing corn. Bathing symbolizes purity and the importance of water. In representing Hopi cultural values, these symbols provide the newborn with a safe passage through childbirth phases by which he or she becomes a Hopi.

When a Cheyenne baby was born, the midwife was assisted by older women who, because of their age, had spiritual sanction to administer herbal medicines to ease delivery (Bancroft-Hunt 1981:46). These older women were able to appeal to sacred powers for guidance and protection of the child. The midwife would tie the afterbirth in a bag, remove it from the camp, and hang it from a tree because the Cheyenne believed that if she buried it the child would die. When it dried, a piece of the umbilical cord was preserved in a small beaded and quilled buckskin pouch, shaped like a turtle, lizard, or snake, to be fastened to the front of the cradle as a plaything. Later, it was fastened to clothing or worn around the neck as a charm to ensure long life. If the baby died a few days after birth or before it was named, it would not be mourned because it was considered a "spirit-child" who had returned to the other world, from whence it would be reborn.

The afterbirth was to be treated with care since it represented once-vital links between the mother and child. It must be dried, preserved, and worn in a pouch shaped like an animal that lives in the water or in the ground, especially in caves—symbolic of the mother's womb. The turtle is also important in Cheyenne origin myths. Birth blood symbolizes the mystery and power of women and figures in the belief in an afterlife and the spirit world. Naming only those who survive past a given time period is an indicator of high infant mortality. Naming is also a rite of passage whereby the infant becomes a person with Cheyenne identity. The Cheyenne example illustrates birth rituals functioning on a cultural level and birth deliveries functioning on a biological level—the latter a passage from the womb to the earth and the former a passage from nonculture to culture.

In sum, childbirth is an extraordinary event that involves physiological, social, and cosmological dimensions that are divided into phases which are expressed symbolically. Traditional midwives deal with these aspects in culturally specific ways that are meaningful to the mother and family (Cosminsky 1974; Neumann et al. 1974:24; Paul 1975; Paul and Paul 1975; Sargent 1974). In training midwives, these aspects need to be reinforced in accord with cultural expectations of the community and the physiological well-being of the mother and child. Frequently, health educators are concerned exclusively with physiological dimensions, as if the body was an isolated biomedical entity. Andeans, as do many other people, perceive of their bodies as being related to society and the cosmos.

Educators, nonetheless, must change practices that are detrimental to the health of the mother and child either by replacing the maladaptive practice with one that is healthy as well as culturally acceptable or by modifying the practice so it is no longer harmful. This implies the need for an a priori understanding of the culture; skills in cross-cultural communication and teaching; an interest or desire to respect and work within the cultural milieu of the midwives, TBAs and their patients; and a willingness to allow patients some control over their lives and the medical care they receive.

Selection of Individuals to Be Trained as Midwives

Selection Criteria. In the procedure of selecting candidates for midwife training, the focus is often on whether to choose young women, who are more likely to be able to read and write and who will live longer and thus provide a greater return for the investment made in their training, or older women, who possess accumulated wisdom and have the community's respect. Although youth and literacy are advantageous in the retention of instructive material and the ability to keep records (Ampofo et al. 1977:201–3; Neumann et al. 1974:23), limiting the training to the young and literate serves more as a function of easing the trainer's and supervisor's work than serving the community and its real and perceived needs.

With training techniques that rely less on lectures and written material and more on visual aids (demonstrations, posters, projects, and slides) and participant interaction (sociodramas, role playing, and group discussion), literacy becomes less important in the acquisition of knowledge. This was the case in Indonesia, where semiliterate TBAs were trained to enter maternal risk factors on a simple prenatal record card (Alisjahbana et al. 1986:240–42); in Bangladesh (Khan et al. 1985), where illiterate TBAs kept records with the help of literate friends or neighbors; and in Papua New Guinea (Schumacher 1987), in Nicaragua, Central America (Morelli and Missoni 1986), and in Ghana, West Africa (Ampofo et al. 1977), where role playing, demonstrations, and discussions replaced lectures and readings. In India, trainers drew sketches of the designated use on bottles of drugs that were to be administered by the midwives, and then the midwives were made familiar with the smell and color of the bottle's contents through repeated exercises (Dwivedi and Rai 1971).

Both young and old candidates should receive training in order to provide continuity for younger apprentices and to utilize the knowledge and leadership of older midwives. These older midwives should be allowed the opportunity to assist in training the younger ones, serving as special cultural consultants, in order to avoid potential animosity by preserving the community's hierarchy of apprenticeship (see Schumacher 1987).

Selection criteria should be flexible in order to meet the needs of the community and its health programs. For example, a training program in Nicaragua required the following of the applicant:

> The candidate must live in the community and be accepted as a TBA.... She must have at least two years' experience in birth attendance and have helped with at least five deliveries within the past year. She needs to accept the rules laid down by the Ministry of Health and must be willing to attend a training course. Age limits are based on the judgment of the staff responsible for the course. However, these criteria are sometimes adapted to fit the individual case. After a candidate is chosen, the trainer visits her home to get an idea of the midwife's personality and her hygiene. (Morelli and Missoni 1986:146).

In Oruro, Bolivia, candidates were required to work land in the community as an indication of stability. This was because the previously chosen trainees, who were without land, had eventually migrated to the city, taking their upgraded skills with them.

Community Participation. Whatever criteria are used, it is essential to involve community members in the selection of those they think are most appropriate and devoted to providing quality health care (Dwivedi and Rai 1971). In the Department of Oruro, approximately one-third of the community health workers (CHWs) are midwives. Community selection eases the attrition rate experienced by programs that unilaterally recruit midwives. Midwives not selected by the community are, in general, marginally concerned with community life and may be more interested in obtaining positions within the Ministry of Health than serving the local population. They frequently move out of the community or quit practicing once they realize that there is little monetary compensation.

Recruiting from within the community also ensures that the candidates will have a personal link with their clients, will observe the proper modes of conduct, will be fluent in the local dialect, and will know the local etiology of illness. Midwives who are already active within and respected by a community are the ones who should be trained to upgrade their skills. Their selection eliminates conflicts between locally approved midwives and foreign but technically skilled midwives who have not yet gained the confidence of the village mothers. The selection of respected midwives can be done by asking members of the community who they are. Also, if families have health records, there should be an entry for the midwife or TBA who delivered a baby, and these records would identify the popular ones. Local recruitment insures the midwife's ability to provide the additional necessary services integral to her profession, such as cooking ritual meals, washing the mother's clothes, proper handling of the placenta and umbilicus, and conducting prescribed rituals and ceremonies.

Recruitment from within the community is also an opportune time to prepare the people for innovations and to alleviate attendant fears. A common procedure in Latin America is to ask the *Comité de Salud* (Health Committee) to assemble the community and supervise the election of candidates. At these meetings, health problems concerning pregnancy and child care are discussed in order to arrive at some common solutions. If community members are sufficiently concerned, they are asked to elect a midwife for training. If after training the midwife, the community and the *Comité de Salud* determine that she is not carrying out her responsibilities, they may petition the Ministry of Health to remove her, and they then select another candidate. Community preparedness and decision making are crucial to the success of articulated midwifery programs that ask the local midwives to work with the Ministry of Health or local doctors (Neumann et al. 1974:24).

Dr. Abraham Mariaca, an obstetrician, described a case in Kaata, Bolivia, in which a Kallawaya woman had a breech delivery. Her family refused to call Dr. Mariaca because she did not want to be examined and delivered by a male doctor. The *manteo* was employed to try to reposition the baby, but this made matters worse. When the baby's arm protruded first, a midwife amputated it to save the mother's life. Mariaca was called but it was too late; the mother and child bled to death. Mariaca subsequently recommended that a female obstetrician be stationed in the region. Although cases like this are rare, they point out the need for specialists, both midwives and obstetricians, to be able to work together within the cultural predispositions of the community.

Training of Midwives and TBAs

Many midwives and TBAs live in remote and relatively inaccessible areas, and they are often unaware that the government may think they need to upgrade their skills. Furthermore, they are busy raising families and farming, and attendance at training courses often imposes hardships on their families. Trainers need to convince midwives and members of their community of the importance of additional training (Dwivedi and Rai 1971; Neumann et al. 1974:21). However, it is unrealistic to send a letter from the Ministry of Health in the provincial city to a small remote rural village and expect the midwife to show up at the training session.

Training sessions must be at locations easily accessible to the midwives, preferably in rural communities, away from the distractions of the city. And the sessions should be short; two weeks are usually the most that midwives can be absent from their homes. A series of two-week courses should be programmed over several years to progressively educate the midwives. This provides an opportunity for periodic evaluation of their performance, with the possibility of modifying their practice and improving the pedagogy of the trainer. After each course, midwives should be assigned certain procedures, such as aseptic treatment of the umbilical cord, to practice in the interim before the next course. Only if the midwives do their homework should they be allowed to attend subsequent courses.

Cross-Cultural Communication. The keys to successful midwife training are the trainers. The most successful trainers are natives of the culture, fluent in the popular language, and knowledgeable in ethno- and biomedicine. They are also patient, enthusiastic, and never condescending. In Bolivia, doctors and technicians are frequently poor trainers because of their overbearing attitudes and scientific prejudices. The best trainers have been people educated in medical anthropology, cross-cultural communication, and public health and who have experience in working with midwives. There is no substitute for educators who have a deep love for the peasants and are motivated to improve their health.

A basic training program for midwives and TBAs includes instruction on prenatal nutrition, prenatal screening for potential problems (see Alisjahbana et al. 1986:240–42; Janowitz et al. 1985), methods of aseptic delivery and cord treatment, pre- and postpartum nutritional counseling, and family planning. Effective counseling includes information on necessary nutrients, what available foods contain these nutrients, and the importance of breast-feeding and colostrum. Oral rehydration therapy for infants with diarrhea needs to become second nature for midwives, TBAs, and mothers.

Handling Complications. Prenatal screening to detect problems is difficult in areas where TBAs are involved only in the delivery process and where clinics are inaccessible. The best solution is one in which TBAs and midwives diagnose the problem well in advance so that the mother is transported to a clinic when it becomes necessary. But in remote areas and in emergencies, midwives and TBAs need to be trained to deal with such problems. Educators need to emphasize, however, that these measures are only to be used in emergencies and that early diagnosis and treatment with specialists are preferred. Educators also need to weigh the ethical dilemma of having the midwife intervene in an extraordinary way during an emergency and perhaps complicate matters or having her wait for help, a delay that might result in the death of the mother and her baby.

In Sierra Leone, Africa, the maternal mortality rate due to ante- and postpartum hemorrhage is very high. It was decided to train midwives to administer oral ergometrine, which causes uterine contractions within six-and-a-half to eight minutes, and to manually remove the unexpelled placenta (Aitken et al. 1985). In India, doctors provide midwives with a kit containing nutritional supplements, 100 tablets of iron and folic acid, and two doses of tetanus toxoid injections (Pratinidhi et al. 1985).

Visual Aids. In Nicaragua, educators train midwives to use a kit containing the following items: a plastic mat to be put under the mother, a plastic apron to be worn by the midwife, scissors and forceps, thread to bind the cord and iodine-alcohol to disinfect the stump, tetracycline ophthalmic cream, two towels, soap, a scrub brush for hands and nails, and cotton wool and gauze. The midwives learn how to give intramuscular injections and identify complications for referral to clinics by using cards with pictures. After marking the suspected complication by tearing off a section of the card, the midwife sends the mother to the clinic with the card (Morelli and Missoni 1986:147).

Nicaraguan educators teach midwives in simple language rich in popular expressions and with visual aids. Some of the visual aids are aprons with a normal and pregnant uterus painted on them which are worn by the midwives to explain basic anatomy to the mother, a doll with colored strings attached to represent the newborn and its umbilical cord's arteries and veins, and a piece of cloth to represent the placenta. They avoid medical or scientific terms, graphs, and texts. Because the midwives are older women with little literacy, this pedagogy is effective (Morelli and Missoni 1986).

In Bolivia, Ghana, and Huon Peninsula, health evaluators report the effective use of role-playing, models, and drawings in training sessions (Bastien 1987:77–85; Ampofo et al. 1977:200; Schumacher 1987:214). In Bolivia, role-playing is particularly effective in training candidates to understand the other person's point of view. For example, midwives play the role of nurse and doctors play the role of midwife. After each role-playing session, the trainees discuss ways to improve their performances. Acting out is an excellent way to remember what they have learned.

After the midwives complete the training course in Bolivia, they are honored in a graduation program that includes diplomas, speeches, and a celebration. The prestige gained by completing the course is motivational for them. Providing the graduates with delivery kits will assist them technically in their practice, but the presentation also serves as a ritual signifying newly acquired knowledge.

Unsuccessful Results. The director of Project Concern in Oruro, Grisel Saenz, discontinued training midwives for the Department of Oruro because their performance was unsatisfactory. The Ministry of

Health and Project Concern considered the training program ineffective because those whom they had trained did not collaborate
fully with doctors and nurses, did not adopt biomedical practices,
and had little effect on decreasing child mortality. Grisel maintained
that because in rural communities there were so many traditional
birth attendants, from the husband to the grandmother, it was
impossible to distinguish the TBAs from the midwives. As a result,
TBAs were frequently trained instead of those who were more active
in the profession. Nonetheless, Grisel reported considerable success
in training community health workers who also act as midwives.

Project Concern and the Ministry of Health did little to support
the midwives after their training. There was no association formed
for them as there was for the CHWs; there were no supplementary
courses, and no ongoing supervision. Furthermore, the directors
had difficulty organizing the midwives, who are uniquely independent and set in their ways. The inflexibility of the midwives and the
bureaucracy of the Ministry of Health hampered its capability to
find a culturally sensitive approach to their training. After inter-
viewing midwives trained in the program, Oscar Velasco (pers. com.
1989) found that midwives complained that the procedures they
were taught had caused their clientele to decrease in size and that
one midwife had lost so many patients that she stopped practicing
altogether.

The failure of midwife training in Oruro does not support Grisel's or others' argument for the discontinuation of training midwives. Rather it shows the need (1) to articulate biomedicine with
ethnomedicine in the training of midwives, (2) to educate members
of the community about changes expected of the midwife and to rely
on its members to select midwives who would serve their needs, (3) to
outfit midwives with culturally appropriate equipment, (4) to assist
them in forming associations independent of the biomedical establishment but collaborating with it, and (5) to provide ongoing training courses and supervision.

Family Planning

Spacing Births. Midwives and TBAs need to be trained to provide
counsel and aid in the implementation of family planning because
they are important in the integration of family planning and maternal and child health in developing countries. Family planning, sometimes referred to as family spacing, remains a focus of public health
concern for obvious reasons (Neumann et al. 1976; Mull 1990:35). The

time interval for population doubling in the poorest countries ranges from 16 to 50 years, as compared with 100 years for most Western nations and 1,000 years for Sweden. Thus the poorest countries literally outgrow their own successes in agriculture and economics; and many are getting poorer year after year (Bell and Reich 1988). Where the average birth interval is less than two years, infant mortality is usually high (Hobcraft et al. 1983; Morley and Lovel 1986:112; Mull 1990:35). Nevertheless, reasons for family planning may not be so obvious to some doctors in Bolivia who take a pronatalist point of view and see a positive *nationalistic* element in a high birth rate (Timothy Wright, pers. com. 1992).

Family planning does not restrict having the number of children a couple desires. It simply provides a means to space births, delay childbearing until the woman or couple is ready, or stop bearing children after the family is considered complete. Forced sterilization is unethical, and its use in controlling birth rates has backfired, as in the cases of Bolivia by USAID and the Peace Corps during the 1950s and 1960s and in India under Indira Gandhi. In both countries, women were sterilized without their knowledge. This procedure caused subsequent mistrust of health programs. Also, care should be taken to ensure that family planning is not perceived as a coercive measure, so that couples will actively participate in deciding what is best for them and not resist the information and services being offered.

The Opposition. In most countries where there is opposition to family planning, it is usually due to religious and political issues. In Bolivia, for example, designers of a Child Survival Program (1990–1995) had to be careful not to include family planning lest some Bolivians perceive of this as opposition to Catholicism and a form of United States imperialism that would limit the one asset the poor have: their children.

If objections to family planning are raised, trainers need to teach midwives how to answer them. Objections are often based on ignorance and rumors. In Bolivia, women refused to be vaccinated with tetanus toxoid because they had heard that this would sterilize them, and others said that milk products donated by Food for Peace contained sterilization chemicals. These rumors are difficult to disprove. Ironically, Dr. Oscar Velasco conducted a study of why women received tetanus toxoid shots and found that some did it because they believed it did sterilize them. Also, Bastien learned in his work with Kallawaya herbalists that women frequently requested herbs for family planning, both to conceive and to prevent pregnancy. One observation is that those who object to family planning are men, mestizos, and politicians. Peasant women in Bolivia want it as an option and continually ask for help in planning their families.

The Advantages. Although the issue can be a sensitive one, any program designed to upgrade maternal and child health must include family planning. Birth spacing of at least two years increases maternal and infant survivability, and reduces morbidity when other factors such as endemic disease are present. The health of mothers and children is influenced by family size, or, more accurately, by birth spacing (Hobcraft et al. 1983; Morley and Lovel 1986:112; Mull 1990:35). If there are at least two years between pregnancies, the mother is better able to recoup her own physiological losses, and children have a greater chance of being well cared for, of being breast-fed longer, and of being taller and heavier. Thus, birth spacing can reduce considerably the infant mortality rate.

Due to the type of bonds midwives usually form with their patients, and because the nature of their work deals with birth and infant care, midwives can be an invaluable work force for the dissemination and collection of family-planning information (Cosminsky 1977:100). Before training midwives, educators should assess the need for family planning by a survey interview regarding morbidity and mortality, as well as the receptiveness to family planning. One such survey was conducted by members of the Danfa team in Ghana (Belcher et al. 1975; 1978).

Multiple Pregnancies = Multiple Deaths. Many women are motivated by social pressure to be sexually active and to have many children. Bolivians do not understand the relationship between family planning and maternal and child health. More research on sexual behavior and attitudes is needed to study the interplay between social pressure to have many children (or not have many) and social pressure to be sexually active. Since intercourse is consensual, frequent pregnancies are not viewed as being problematic. But if infants are spaced too closely together, the mothers are forced to wean them early, which places a severe nutritional stress on the infant. Where infant mortality is high, couples continue to have children as insurance that some will survive to support them, creating a spiraling cycle of maternal and infant morbidity and mortality. In areas where infant mortality has decreased, thus reducing the need for this rea-

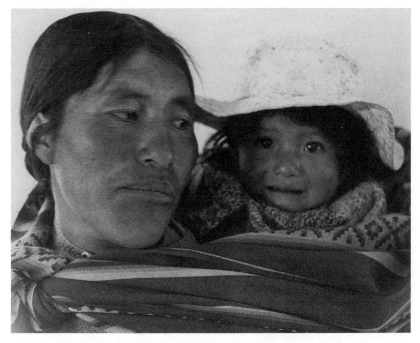

Aymara mother and child. Many mothers want family planning, but their husbands disapprove.

soning, couples desire contraceptive strategies (Mandelbaum 1974; Stycos 1968).

In Asia, one-fourth and, in Latin America, one-half of maternal deaths are attributed to complications resulting from abortion. The World Fertility Survey for 1980–81 estimated that 300 million couples in Africa and Asia did not want more children but that they were not using birth-control measures (Sai et al. 1986:316, 320).

Multiple pregnancies increase the incidences of malnutrition, morbidity, birth complications, and economic hardship. They can debilitate the mother, making her susceptible to anemia, a complication estimated to be responsible for 40 to 50 percent of the maternal deaths in the developing world (Sai et al. 1986:316), as well as such endemic diseases as malaria in Africa and tuberculosis in the Andean countries of South America. A pregnant or lactating mother is less able to work than before and therefore contributes less to the family income, reinforcing the cycle of malnutrition, morbidity, and mortality. Indirect causes, such as the above, account for about one-fourth of the maternal deaths worldwide (Sai et al. 1986:316, 320).

Education = Self-Determination. A key to successful family-planning programs is to allow people to determine how many children they would like to have and then provide the education and services necessary for them to act according to their decisions. Overemphasizing contraception can cause the members of the community to reject other health measures. For instance, in Nicaragua, midwives advocated birth control so adamantly that they were associated with limiting life, a role that community members could not tolerate. Planners readjusted the emphasis to support the more traditional practices of midwives, who became consultants rather than advocates for family planning (Morelli and Missoni 1986:144). In Tegucigalpa, Honduras, USAID directs a project where pills and condoms are distributed through one or two women in each rural community. There has been some success in that the women use the pill but the men refuse to use the condoms (Libbett Crandon-Malamud, pers. com. 1990). The women were able to distribute the pills to other women in the community.

Because men must be active in the decision to use birth control for it to be an acceptable and effective recourse, sex education for men is as essential as it is for women. Men, however, frequently oppose family planning: they do not use condoms and they actively resist birth control throughout the world. An effective way to deal with this is to train male midwives. Although many project planners view birth assistance as a feminine-controlled activity, this is not true cross-culturally. For example: the male midwives among the Aymara of the Department of Oruro.

If male and female midwives are trained to aid in the implementation of family planning, they need to be provided with contraceptives and the skills to administer them. Brigitte Jordan (1978:58) reports an incident where a midwife was trained in contraception but was supplied only two packets of birth-control pills. Some methods of birth control, such as intrauterine devices or injectables, require technical skills that can be learned by midwives. Inayatullah in Sai et al. (1986:328) writes that oral contraceptives, condoms, and spermicides are particularly suited to community-based systems, but "barrier methods" (condoms and diaphragms) require high motivation and consistency, and the pill requires multiple visits to doctors.

The Norplant method offers great promise as an effective and long-term birth-control method for peoples throughout the world. Doctors implant six inch-long silicone capsules filled with progestin below the surface of the skin underneath the arm in the tricep muscle. Lasting fifteen minutes, the surgery is done with a local anesthetic. Birth control is effective twenty-four hours after implantation for 98.9 to 99.2 percent of the women for five years. In a reverse procedure, capsules can be removed if women wish to conceive. Although Norplant has a proven record in Europe since the 1960s, the FDA only approved its use in the United States in January 1992. Consequently, health workers in the United States have infrequently used Norplant for primary health-care programs in developing countries. Norplant is costly: in the Dallas–Forth Worth area, doctors in private clinics charge from $700 to $1,200 and those in family-planning clinics from no cost to $500. Nonetheless, for peoples of developing countries with skyrocketing populations, the initial cost of Norplant is well worth the long-term birth control that it provides. Moreover, after implantation, Norplant requires nothing to take, inject, clean, and maintain. (Hatcher et al. 1992:301–31).

Similar to Norplant, Depo-Provera are injections of progestin that provide birth control for three or six months. Slightly more effective than Norplant, one woman out of 400 stands a risk of pregnancy in a year. Because Depo-Provera requires return visits to doctors, it is less suitable than Norplant.

In areas where technical, economic, religious, or political factors have restricted the use of contraceptives, natural forms such as prolonged breast-feeding and rhythm methods (avoidance of intercourse during peak fertility cycles) can be employed at a low cost, but with a limited rate of success (Sai et al. 1986:331).

Compensation, Licenses, Certification, and Supervision

Major issues to consider when integrating midwives and TBAs into health programs are compensation, certification, and supervision. Midwives who have completed courses and are contributing to health care should be publicly recognized, respected, and legitimized by doctors and nurses. The type of compensation for attending births, however, is better left to the discretion of the community, as has been the custom. This avoids resentments that might arise from paying someone who traditionally provided a service for the good of the community without monetary compensation or overpaying someone who provides services considered comparable to another person's services.

Community Support. When selecting candidates, educators can inform members of the community that the midwife will not be paid by the government and that it is the community's responsibility to compensate her. As in the case with community health workers, salaries for midwives are also discouraged because of the cost to governments already in debt and subject to economic crises. Midwife training programs should enable the community to be nearly autonomous, permitting members of the community, rather than outside agencies and the government, to be responsible for their own health and health needs.

Licensing. The issue of licensing is complex. To a large extent, the degree of licensing provided should depend on the level of training the midwife received and her degree of accountability to or autonomy from the governing agency. Licensing does not ensure quality health care, although it can protect the practitioner from spurious lawsuits. In 1983, 82 percent of the countries of the world had training programs for midwives as opposed to 37 percent in 1972. This increase toward their incorporation into the health-care system shows the growing importance of the question of liability for midwives who may perform beyond their abilities, injure a patient due to neglect, or perform an illegal procedure, such as abortion or female circumcision (Owen et al. 1983:291). Litigation is unlikely when the midwife is responsible to the community, whose members have the authority to select and dismiss her with the backing of the Ministry of Health.

It is possible that licensing might be used to restrict the selection of valuable candidates and provide an oppressive mechanism to manipulate or impinge upon the midwive's duties and culture-specific skills (Karim 1984:165). To avoid the abuse of licensing as a means of oppression, it should be reserved for only those midwives who have already reached a level of professionalism such that they seek the protection it would provide.

Certification. Certification indicates a higher level of training and expertise than licensure and is an appropriate means of rewarding and ackowledging the extra effort that midwives have made to upgrade their skills. A method for certification would not make it illegal for the untrained to be active, but it would provide the better trained with some advertisement of their skills (Morelli and Missoni 1986:147). Certification also provides the patients with additional knowledge about the midwife, allowing them to make a better, more informed decision regarding their health care. As the success of training programs becomes evident through increased maternal and child health, it is likely that more mothers will chose certified midwives. Midwives and TBAs look upon certification as a reward for attending courses, and a degree of certification can be issued upon graduating from each of the courses.

Supervision. Supervision is the key to continual improvement of the midwives' skills and their successful integration into health programs (Ampofo et al. 1977; Neumann et al. 1974). Several months after graduation from the training course and periodically thereafter, midwives should be visited by a supervisor, preferably a trainer or a nurse responsible for maternal care in the region. For successful communication and exchange between the supervisor and the midwife, the role of supervisor must not be that of an authoritarian, but instead someone who evaluates, assists, and supports. A supervisor can encourage and motivate the midwife to follow practices learned in the training course. Emphasis throughout the training course should be made that enhancement of the midwife's skills is a long process that only begins with the courses and continues with practice and supervision. All too frequently midwives have been trained and later abandoned without supervision and support, which made their long-term integration into the health program impossible.

Conclusions

Midwives and TBAs are invaluable resources for the upgrading of maternal and child health. They are the most available and widespread of ethnomedical practitioners. Without their assistance, mother and child survival, primary health care, and family-planning programs are unlikely to succeed.

Although many countries have adopted training programs for midwives and TBAs, they have not been as successful as planned for a number of reasons: conflict between the newly trained and the traditional midwives, adoption of inappropriate and maladaptive health practices, little consideration for the community's real and perceived needs, lack of community participation, ignoring cultural beliefs and practices, and lack of training supervision.

Ethnographic studies are necessary to evaluate the needs of the community and detect potential problems that could occur. Selection of candidates, course content, method of training, and remuneration will be dependent on the needs, real and perceived, of each community.

If midwives and TBAs are to be integrated into health programs, doctors and nurses must respect them for their skills and knowledge of indigenous customs and resources, as well as support and encourage them in the practice of their craft.

PART IV
Doctors, Nurses, and Vaccinators

STRATEGIES FOR JOINT THERAPIES

7

Training Doctors to Integrate Ethnomedicine

Bolivian doctors and nurses are beginning to collaborate with ethnomedical practitioners (see Bastien 1982a). The following example provides a case in point. A father and mother brought their fifteen-year-old daughter to Dr. Oscar Velasco for consultation, saying that she had nausea, fainting spells, and nervous tics. After examining her, Velasco realized that she was pregnant. (The daughter had attended a fiesta, gotten drunk, and been raped by a mestizo.) However, he didn't mention the pregnancy because she was unmarried, and he feared her parents would whip her and consider the child illegitimate. Instead, he referred them to a diviner who was informed of the situation. This diviner had cured several patients in cooperation with Velasco. The diviner performed an elaborate ritual with the young woman and her relatives present. Divining from the coca leaves, he said that she had risen during the middle of the night to urinate outside, and as she was doing so, *Pachamama* (Mother Earth) had impregnated her with a child.

The father became furious on hearing that his daughter was pregnant, but was unable to do much because the diviner had structured the behavior and illness within a ritual and social context. When the diviner continued throwing the coca leaves, he inferred that the father had been involved in promiscuous activity and therefore should judge himself before his daughter. As the ritual continued, the daughter and her parents became reconciled and offered a llama fetus, coca leaves, and guinea-pig blood to *Pachamama*. Her father said that he would accept the infant into his family and give it his last name.

Aymara and Quechua Indians prefer to deal with illnesses as symbols that make them endurable and acceptable to members of the community. Although some doctors equate these symbols with ignorance, Velasco understood how diviners use symbols and rituals as adaptive mechanisms enabling people to cope with maladies. He also knew that he needed an ethnomedical practitioner to deal with complex behavioral and social problems. This knowledge and collaboration prevented unwarranted suffering and another illegitimate or unaccepted child.

173

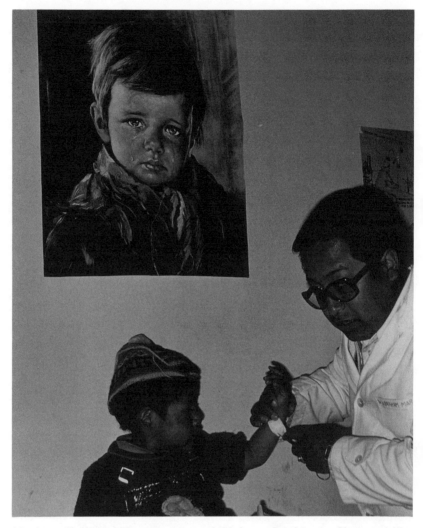

Abraham Mariaca, M.D., treating a child for a dog bite in Charazani. Dr. Mariaca speaks both Aymara and Quechua and was well-loved by the Kallawaya. He was forced to discontinue practicing at the hospital by middle-class mestizos because he identified with peasants.

Workshops for Biomedical and Ethnomedical Practitioners

Once doctors and nurses in the Department of Oruro, Bolivia, became aware of how the symbols and rituals of ethnomedical practices function within Andean culture, they were better able to relate to patients' needs and feelings and to cooperate with practitioners.

This collaboration between biomedical and ethnomedical practitioners was a result of workshops in which doctors and nurses, together with ethnomedical practitioners, shared information about illnesses, frequently perceived in cultural, biological, and social terms. At the level of suffering and sickness, biomedical and ethnomedical practitioners have much to share with one another, and these workshops provided this opportunity.

Workshops linking bio- and ethnomedicine for government health personnel are effective provided the participants are given appropriate cross-cultural training, with specific emphasis on the beliefs and practices of ethnomedicine (Neumann and Lauro 1982). The Ministry of Rural Health in Oruro and Project Concern initiated these workshops, which have since been effective and can be used as a model for coordinated health planning in other parts of the world. Dr. Oscar Velasco, Angela Lutena, and I worked with diviners, herbalists, midwives, and other ethnomedical practitioners to conduct these workshops. The objectives of the workshops were education of biomedical practitioners in ethnomedicine, instruction of ethnomedical practitioners in biomedicine, strategies for collaboration, and unified action for a child-survival program that involves community participation and ethnomedical practitioners.

The workshops were five days long, and about twelve of them were given between 1981 and 1985. After 1985 they were continued sporadically. The participants were directors of the Ministry of Health, doctors, nurses, community health workers, anthropologists, midwives, shamans, diviners, and technicians (agronomists, vaccinators, and social workers). The workshops were held in rural communities, usually market centers, that were accessible to ethnomedical practitioners. We slept and ate in *pensiones* (hostels) and met at the community center for the discussions. We tried to conduct the workshops as close to peasant life as possible, avoiding undue association with the dominant medical establishment. Collegiality was encouraged by dances, parties, and sharing food. Field trips to agricultural extension services, archaeological sites, and clinics were scheduled.

Joint therapy sessions were important during the workshops, and if patients were not available, individuals substituted for them by role-playing. Demonstrations of curing rituals were presented by ethnomedical practitioners with doctors and nurses as participants. Upon completion of a workshop, participants were given elegant diplomas, a banquet, and some practical medical aid: doctors were given medicinal plants, community health workers received herbal

manuals and first-aid kits, and midwives were given kits for sterilizing instruments. The participants enjoyed the workshops and frequently returned the next year.

Correspondences between Medicines

One outcome of the workshops was that biomedical and ethnomedical practitioners were able to draw correspondences between experiences of illnesses. They were able to zero in on particular joint
strategies for improving health. Doctors soon realized that ethnomedical practitioners used adaptive and popular strategies for curing which peasants readily accepted. Ethnomedical practitioners
became aware of public health measures and medicines that could
help their patients and members of the community. They were also
interested in rural and community development projects discussed
during the workshops, such as solar gardens, latrines, and smokeless
ovens.

Another outcome was that ethnomedical practitioners helped us
present alternative modes of curing, especially rituals. With their
help we were able to outline the correspondence between culturally
classified illnesses and biomedical pathology so that doctors and
nurses could translate this symbolic language into medical terms
meaningful in their profession (Bastien 1987:77–86).

An Example: Diarrhea. Diarrhea provides an illustration of how biomedical and ethnomedical practitioners arrived at correspondences
in their classification, etiology, and treatment of illnesses. Diarrhea
is the major killer of infants throughout the world, and the majority
die from dehydration. Collaboration between biomedical and ethnomedical practitioners is mandatory in order to convince peasants
to use oral rehydration therapy to stop deaths from diarrhea.

During the workshops, biomedical and ethnomedical practitioners participated in a group session where they listed the names,
symptoms, causes, and treatment of diarrhea in two columns, one
for biomedicine and the other for ethnomedicine. Under ethnomedicine they listed Aymara and Quechua words used to describe
diarrhea: *curso* (flow), *wijch'uy* (expel rapidly, also used for vomiting),
mal de pato (duck disease), *aika* (diarrhea from change), *wila curso* (flow
of blood), and *mancharisqa* (emotional diarrhea, often associated
with *susto*).

Once doctors and nurses became aware that Andeans of Oruro
distinguished between different degrees of diarrhea, they were bet-

ter able to query patients about this and educate them concerning treatment of the various kinds. One doctor observed that ignorance of this had led to a serious mistake by having posters made classifying all diarrhea as *aika* and stating that it was a deadly killer, whereas Aymaras and Quechuas considered it least important, often found in babies and travelers and caused by change of food, lodging, and climate. *Wijch'uy* describes temporary cases of diarrhea, whereas *curso* refers to persistent cases, and *curso wila* to perduring cases with blood in the stool (dysentery). Under biomedicine, doctors and nurses translated the ethnomedical taxonomy into corresponding biomedical terms. They realized that these Andeans classify diarrhea into categories translatable into biomedical pathology and that for this and other sicknesses doctors and nurses should begin by investigating the taxonomy of the disease. (Since therapeutic techniques vary considerably from place to place among ethnomedical practitioners, it is necessary for doctors and nurses along with medical anthropologists to take the time to investigate the native etiology and regional taxonomies. This information could be published as a reference book to be used by health practitioners in the region.)

Once doctors, nurses, and ethnomedical practitioners had compared taxonomies, they respectively listed symptoms, causes, and treatments. They disagreed on symptoms because each type of practitioner was relating diarrhea to different causes. Although ethnomedical practitioners included dehydration as a symptom in other illnesses, they did not associate diarrhea with thirst, sunken eyes, and crying without tears because they believed that diarrhea is a wet disease with wet symptoms. It is not associated with dehydration, but with a surplus of fluids. They also treated diarrhea by further drying the person out with absorbent cereals.

The doctors and nurses explained to the ethnomedical practitioners that this practice furthers the victim's chances of dying from dehydration. The ethnomedical practitioners accepted this by admitting that diarrhea could also be a dry disease. They all agreed that persistent diarrhea was deadly, which was a common experience of biomedical and ethnomedical practitioners in the Andes.

The most creative exchange occurred when doctors, nurses, midwives, herbalists, and diviners agreed upon the use of herbal teas with an adequate amount of sugar and some salt to treat diarrhea. Before the discussion, doctors had promoted the UNICEF rehydration envelopes to treat diarrhea, but these were costly, frequently unavailable, and misleading to patients, who perceived them as cures for diarrhea. (Patients did not distinguish between a rehydration formula and a cure for diarrhea. They felt cheated when, after using the envelopes, the diarrhea continued.) After the herbalists explained how different plants were used to treat the various types of diarrhea, doctors and nurses came to respect this practical knowledge. Even though they still doubted the curative effects of herbal teas, they were more receptive once Oscar Velasco and I explained that plant leaves contain potassium, and that herbal teas with sugar are alternative rehydration formulas which biomedical and ethnomedical practitioners can prescribe and have accepted by peasants, *cholos*, mestizos, and others because Bolivians love to take teas.

Role-Playing and Sociodramas. In these workshops, doctors, nurses, midwives, herbalists, and diviners participated in the diagnosis and treatment of cultural illnesses. In role-playing sessions, peasants presented their symptoms in cultural contexts foreign to the participants, who then had to diagnose and provide therapy. The observers offered suggestions until some understanding was reached. The doctors readily realized their incapacity to relate to Aymara and Quechua patients, who not only spoke foreign languages but also described the symptoms in very diffuse terms. Any ailments within the thorax were described as *chuyma usutu* (my heart aches). Simple procedures used by midwives, such as greeting patients in their native languages and offering them coca leaves, brought much better relationships between patients and doctors. The nurses observed that the peasants were more confident in them if they touched them, as the herbalists did when they treated the patients.

Sociodramas were also used to induce collaboration between biomedical and ethnomedical practitioners. In sociodramas, participants were asked to enact a social setting with some problem, such as a family with a member sick. Both biomedical and ethnomedical practitioners were assigned separately to prepare curing sessions for a culturally defined illness, such as *susto*. The following day they enacted the therapeutic session, some playing the ailing individual and the family, and others playing the herbalist, ritualist, and doctor. The next day, biomedical and ethnomedical practitioners jointly prepared a sociodrama. At first, they were told to enact it according to what they believed usually happens, which enabled the participants and observers to reflect on present practices or lack of articulation. Then they were asked to devise a collaborative and culturally sensitive therapeutic session with herbalists, ritualists, midwives, nurses, and doctors.

Role-playing and sociodramas are effective because they allow

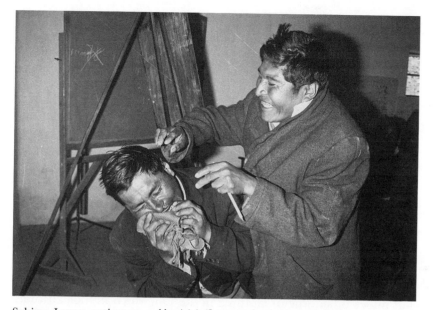

Sabino Lauro acting as a *kharisiri* (fat-snatcher) in a sociodrama to cure *liquichado.*

biomedical and ethnomedical practitioners to do their own anthropological analysis on how to collaborate. Both types of practitioners are participants, observers, and "anthropologists" in the drama. This interlocutory style enables the biomedical and ethnomedical practitioners to observe and modify their systems, rather than having a foreign anthropologist doing this for them. Because both practitioners need to processually devise health planning that is somewhere between biomedicine and ethnomedicine, a discursive or interlocutory process is essential so they can modify each other's views and practices.

Aseptic Campaigns. A major conflict between ethnomedical and biomedical practitioners is that the latter abhors the former's unaseptic practices. Ethnomedical practitioners do not subscribe to the antiseptic and sterile premise of biomedicine because germs are not their major concern. This can be a problem in the clinics. Severo, the nurse in Qaqachaka, removed an herbal compress from a leg injury because it looked unclean and was unable to put on a clean bandage because he didn't have one.

In Achacachi, Joe Picardi campaigned against ethnomedical practitioners because he said that, with unsterile compresses, they caused more infections than they cured. During the 1960s, Kallawayas reported that people treated with herbal remedies were not allowed admission into the American-run Methodist hospital in Ancoraimes. While I was in Kaata in 1971, Kallawayas were preparing an injured person to be taken to the Methodist hospital. They removed the herbal compresses, saying that the doctor would not allow them to enter if the patient had used herbal remedies. The doctor had told them that the use of plants was the work of the devil in the Garden. Whether the doctor said this is questionable; this hospital has maintained a good relationship with ethnomedical practitioners through the years (Libbet Crandon-Malamud, pers. com. 1991).

During the workshops, doctors and nurses educated ethnomedical practitioners about hygiene, infections, and sterility to help them be more effective in their therapy. Ethnomedical practitioners usually carry alcohol for ritual purposes, so the nurses showed them how this can be used to cleanse and disinfect wounds. Lutena and Velasco provided them with sterilizing kits and instructed them to put infected bedding or clothing in the sun, which in high altitudes destroys many microorganisms. Ethnomedical practioners were also instructed on building latrines and given concrete slabs to cover them. At first they objected to defecating inside the earth, which they consider sacred, but resolved this problem by saying that they could construct the latrines in nonsacred places. Doctors and nurses were surprised at the flexibility of ethnomedical practitioners' beliefs in adapting to biomedicine.

Fortunately, Andean people are frequently naturally resistant to microorganisms because they have adapted to conditions not as sterile as those found in developed countries. In general, aseptic campaigns have been ineffective in the Andes because peasants lack toilets, sewage systems, and water to continually cleanse themselves. Even though they have some resistance, malnutrition makes them vulnerable to disease. The nurses and doctors also instructed ethnomedical practioners in first aid, hygiene, pathology, and referral of patients when warranted.

Concerning texts for similar workshops, Kroeger and Luna (1985) edited a guide with simple explanations and appropriate medical technology for doctors and nurses working in rural areas of Latin America. For helping health personnel in matters of cross-cultural communication, Werner and Bower (1982) is useful. For ethnomedical practitioners, David Werner's *Donde No Hay Doctor* (1991), his *Where There Is No Doctor: A Village Health Care Handbook* (1977), Morley and Lovel's *My Name Is Today* (1986), and Phillips's *Health and Health Care in the Third World* (1990) are useful manuals promoting practical, popular health care for developing countries.

Collaboration between Practitioners for Susto

A major objective of the workshops was that doctors and nurses learn the following about cultural illnesses and ethnomedicine: ethnophysiology, etiology, and therapy. From this information, Oscar Velasco prepared a reference manual with body parts, illnesses, and symptoms provided in Aymara, Quechua, and Spanish languages. Doctors and nurses can use this information to recognize cultural illnesses. As a result, doctors are able to collaborate with ethnomedical practitioners, especially regarding culturally defined illnesses.

Collaboration in cases of *susto* illustrates how a culturally defined illness can be jointly treated by biomedical and ethnomedical practitioners. *Susto* (fright) is common in Andean regions and in other parts of Latin America, and it is a cultural illness that needs to be treated jointly by doctors and traditional practitioners (Crandon-Malamud 1983a; Rubel 1964; Rubel et al. 1983, 1984).

Bolivians define *susto* as the loss of *ajayu* or *ánimo*. *Ajayu* is translated as "spirit," but for many Andeans it is associated with emotional fluids that surge from the body because of fright. These fluids are invisible but charged substances similar to electricity that keep the body working. A good scare, such as a charging dog, an assault by a stranger, a scream, or an accident, frightens victims so that they lose their *ajayu*. If the *ajayu* is not recovered, the person dies.

Susto is found most among children and women, mainly because Latin American culture emphasizes *machismo* for adult males, and fearlessness is an indicator of *machismo*. Symptoms of *susto* include somatic disorders, low metabolism, diarrhea, nausea, anorexia, and low fever. Psychological symptoms are depression, melancholy, lack of enthusiasm, withdrawal, nervous tics, staring, and irritability. Any serious personality change may be an indicator of *susto*.

Clinically, Kallawaya herbalists vary in their treatment of *susto*. Mario Salcedo says that it is caused by an alteration within the nervous system. People see things that frighten them so much that their body fluids become sluggish. Bile becomes sludge and blood stops circulating, which causes sicknesses for weak people. Mario treats them with rest, diet, and *matés* of supplejack (*Paullinia cupana* H.B.K.), which is a stimulant like caffeine. He deals with the physical symptoms.

In contrast, Nestor Llaves tries to cure the victim by dealing with the fright and retrieving the *ajayu*. Nestor believes that everybody is prey to *susto*. Next to liver ailments, it is the most commonly recognized illness in Bolivia. (Tuberculosis is the most frequent disease, but Bolivians accept this as a way of life.) Nestor attributes *susto* to psychological and symbolic causes: fright, unrequited love, witchcraft, and the *supay* (a malevolent trickster associated with either the devil or the vengeful dead).

Although *susto* is frequently related to psychological and symbolic factors that are dealt with by ethnomedical practitioners, in Bolivia and in Mexico it is frequently associated with serious illnesses and regarded as an indicator of deep pathological concerns to be treated by biomedical practitioners (Rubel et al. 1983). Both types of treatment can be beneficial simultaneously (Libbet Crandon-Malamud, pers. com. 1990).

Susto has occurred more during times of stress (hyperinflation, high unemployment, and closing of the mines) in Bolivia, but the stress has activated chronic illnesses (Velasco, per. com. 1987). Incidents of *susto* increased among miners of Oruro after companies discontinued tin mining in 1986. Miners were laid off and couldn't find other employment. Oscar Velasco attended a clinic and reported that many miners came to him, reporting that they were *asustado*. They said that they had lost their *ánimo* or *ajayu*. Velasco examined them and found that many were sick with tuberculosis of the throat, kidneys, and of the bile sac in one instance. In a deprived anemic state, these patients were able to endure their illnesses by associating them with *susto*. Losing their jobs added to the stress of poverty, unemployment, and diminishment of role identity and led to increased alcohol consumption. These factors affected the immune system that had once inhibited the tuberculin bacteria. Patients and their families were in crisis.

Diviners and herbalists modified their usual way of treating these patients. Previously, they had been accustomed to curing a patient within one night. After the closure of the mines, they expanded the treatment to last a week or more. They realized that their patients had multiple problems and needed intensive consultation. Collaborating together, doctors assisted the herbalists and diviners by treating the patient and often other members of his family with antibiotics for tuberculosis. Velasco reported successful therapy for many patients when there was collaborative treatment between doctors and herbalists. This indicates that treatment by both doctors and ethnomedical practitioners would be beneficial if used simultaneously in the therapy.

Culturally Defined Illnesses

In those Bolivian hospitals and clinics where collaboration is permitted or arranged, doctors, nurses, diviners, and herbalists combine therapies to treat other culturally defined illnesses related to pathological disorders, such as *lari lari, liquichado,* and *mal de aire.* These experiences provide further illustrations of the need for integrated therapy.

Lari Lari. Peasants of the Department of Oruro believe that *lari lari* is a deadly disease bestowed on victims at night by an owl. Traditional practitioners have elaborate therapies for treating *lari lari* that, alone, are ineffective because it is a symptomatic complex often associated with septicemia. Septicemia is a severe bacteremic infection, generally involving an invasion of the bloodstream by microorganisms in the tissues. Andean infants are susceptible to *lari lari* and many die because the biomedical treatment of septicemia involves intensive care that is not accessible to rural Andeans. *Lari lari* is a cultural illness that necessitates the prompt attention of doctors as well as the collaboration of ethnomedical practitioners.

Mal de Aire. Another cultural illness, *mal de aire* (bad from air), includes muscle and nerve disorders from paralysis, such as Bell's palsy, to muscle cramps. *Mal de aire* is associated with the marasmus theory of disease, or the idea that diseases spread by emanations or vapors ("malaria" derives from *mal de aire*). The marasmus theory is European in origin. Slightly transforming the tropical marasmus theory to the chilly mountainous regions, Bolivians attribute *mal de aire* to the wind *(wayra)*. Herbalists diagnose it as a cold disease that must be cured by hot remedies: steam baths, compresses, and stimulant herbs (coca, anise, and coffee). Mindful of its category, doctors can also prescribe synthetic drugs that coordinate with this system of balancing the hot and cold. For instance, an alcohol massage before an injection or intravenous therapy would associate the injection with a hot remedy (alcohol), making both suitable for *mal de aire,* a cold illness.

Liquichado. As already discussed, Bolivians attribute *liquichado* to the sudden and mysterious removal of fat by a *kharisiri* (cutter). The cutter is usually a doctor, lawyer, or priest who travels at night to remove fat from peasants (Oblitas Poblete 1978:123). The pathological equivalent in biomedicine is tuberculosis. Some herbalists attempt to cure *liquichado* by recommending foods high in fat: soup made from the marrow of burro bones and fat from the pancreas of a sheep. They also perform rituals to regain the fat. These therapies appear effective to Andeans because fat is a principal body fluid associated with energy. For a long time, Andeans referred to a gentleman as a *"wiraqocha"* (sea of fat). Fat provides energy and warmth to Andeans, especially those debilitated by tuberculosis. Apparently, cholesterol is not a problem for Andeans in that they have relatively low incidences of high blood pressure and heart disease. This is also explained by the aerobic effect of working at high altitudes. Respiratory illnesses, together with hypoxia, account for the majority of illnesses, with tuberculosis, pneumonia, and influenza accounting for most deaths.

Herbalists also treat *liquichado* and tuberculosis with diet and rest, which sometimes inhibit the tuberculin bacteria. The patient is "cured" until the next relapse, which involves another healing session. Because tuberculosis is so difficult to cure, herbalists are ineffective in treating it, but they assist patients in adapting to it. Florentino Alvarez continued to treat the disease with rest and diet, as did physicians in Europe and the United States before the discovery of penicillin. One ethnomedical cure is to eat a lizard a day for one year. Doctors use this particular treatment as a precedent in teaching peasants the need to take antibiotic tablets daily for one year, the frequently proscribed biomedical therapy for tuberculosis in Bolivia.

The association of tuberculosis with a *kharisiri* presents an obstacle to ethnomedical practitioners in collaborating with doctors for its treatment because doctors, especially surgeons, are sometimes called *"kharisiris"* ("cutters") and "fat snatchers." The following case, which I observed in Qaqachaka in mid-1982, illustrates the frustration that biomedical practitioners experience in dealing with tuberculin-*kharisiri* patients.

Marcelino, twenty-five years old, had been sick for a year. He had a high fever, was weak, and walked with crutches. The auxiliary nurse, Severo, had diagnosed the disease as tuberculosis of the kidneys, and he had treated Marcelino with antibiotics. When Marcelino felt better, he discontinued taking the pills. Three weeks later, Marcelino became seriously ill. His mother, the village shaman, and the mayor of Qaqachaka, thinking I was a doctor, asked that I cure him. The nurse and I told them that Marcelino was dying, that he needed to be hospitalized in Challapata (three hours by jeep), and that we would take him.

The shaman, Zacarias Chiri, claimed that Marcelino was a victim of the *kharisiri*. Marcelino and members of his family, especially his mother, agreed, and he recalled that someone had removed his fat with an *aparato* (apparatus) while he was traveling (partially intoxicated from chicha) in the bed of a truck through a mestizo community. Because he was in an intoxicated slumber, he could not recall how this was done. Zacarias treated Marcelino with the soup described above. At first, Marcelino recovered; but he suffered a relapse several months later when he became intoxicated from chicha. Zacarias recommended another ritual for that evening and transporting Marcelino to the hospital in the morning.

After three hours' discussion, the mother refused to let her son be taken to the hospital, even though Zacarias recommended it, because she feared he would die there alone. She wanted him to be with his family. Moreover, she also rejected the therapy of Zacarias as the village shaman and said that her husband would bring another, more powerful shaman from a neighboring village. As a possibility, I also think that she associated the physician in the Challapata hospital with "fat snatching" and that she didn't want to put her son in the hands of someone who was associated with the attributed cause of his sickness.

That evening, a visiting shaman prescribed more fat for Marcelino's diet and performed a *turka* ritual (described in chapter 4 in which he went into a trance to talk with Mother Earth, the Dead (Supay), and the Condor. He scolded and punished these deities for taking Marcelino's fat and for trying to take his life. In exchange, he agreed to send them llama fat *(llampu)* and other ritual items. At dawn, he distributed llama fat to the principal earth shrines around the community. His efforts proved ineffectual, and Marcelino died shortly after.

In retrospect, I can see one solution would have been to have the doctor visit and treat Marcelino with the shaman and members of the family present so that they could observe the treatment. One result from the death of Marcelino has been to encourage nurses to treat tuberculosis patients in their homes or within the context of the family. Another has been to offer accommodations for family members in clinics, which can be inexpensively done by providing a

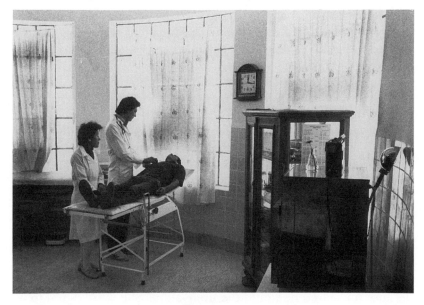

Doctor and nurse attending a Quechua-speaking peasant in a hospital in Department of Cochabamba. Patients do not like being separated from their families and they dislike sterile, white interiors.

mattress, a table, and a cooking stove. In fact, the medical cost is lowered because the family cooks for, washes, and attends the sick person.

In Oruro, Project Concern and the Ministry of Rural Health are raising funds for an integrated hospital with "appropriate technology." The plans call for an adobe hospital without standard metal beds, but with platforms where Andeans can sleep, as in their huts. There will be a room for the patient and another for the family members, where they can cook, eat, and sleep. This follows the practice of herbalists who rarely separate patients from their families.

Through collaboration, Bolivian doctors and nurses are beginning to realize that ethnomedical practitioners and peasants mistrust certain aspects of biomedicine, such as vaccinations, surgery, taking blood, and requiring women to remove their clothes before an examination. With earned trust, sensitivity, flexibility, and creativity, however, they are able to dispel these fears.

At a 1985 symposium in Oruro of doctors, nurses, and ethnomedical practitioners, it was discovered that the *chullpa* illness is sometimes a cultural expression of poliomyelitis and osteomyelitis.

Chullpa is attributed to digging near the graves of ancestors, and its symptoms are protrusions of bone slivers and festering sores.

Sharing Perceptions Cross-Culturally. *Susto, lari lari, liquichado,* and *mal de aire* are a few examples from Bolivia of culturally perceived illnesses. Throughout the world there are many more of these "illness realities" that are expressed in symptomatic complexes, symbols, and bizarre classification systems. Patients perceive the reality of diseases within these categories, which traditional practitioners are able to decipher. But practitioners of biomedicine have little patience for these "smoke screens" that tend to block them from the pathogenic cause of the disease. It is at this juncture that ethnomedical practitioners in Bolivia have assisted doctors and nurses the most in an integrated health program.

These four examples serve to illustrate that the symbols and classification of illnesses constitute a culturally complex system that necessitates the sharing of perceptions among biomedical and ethnomedical practitioners. Practitioners need to advise one another on what are the acceptable therapies, given the cultural classification and scientific evidence. For example, doctors need to inform herbalists that providing diarrhea patients with "dry" remedies is harmful and that rehydration solutions should be given. Diviners need to advise doctors on how to deal with accusations of being a *kharisiri.*

Evaluation of Workshops

Evaluation of the effects of the workshops five years later in 1989 has revealed that the majority of doctors in Oruro have cooperated little with ethnomedical practitioners, but are more understanding of cultural illnesses and accepting of these practitioners. Admittedly, they saw this as one way to increase their practices. More encouraging, a group of five doctors and nurses now actively promote ethnomedicine. They have supported symposia on traditional medicine in Oruro, Cochabamba, and Potosí, Bolivia. Two doctors now collaborate in a clinic with a diviner and herbalist, and a third has adopted the practice of using natural remedies. The Ministry of Rural Health in Oruro established a health post and a director of traditional medicine to stimulate collaboration between ethnomedical and biomedical practitioners. As the first director, Oscar Velasco began regularly to stock medicinal plants in the pharmacy of the Ministry of

Health in Oruro. He later moved to Potosí, where he is currently integrating bio- and ethnomedicine. The present director is Dr. Betty de Soto, who started an integrated hospital in Oruro. Drs. de Soto and Velasco agree that collaboration is slow but that doctors and nurses are changing their attitude from complete rejection of ethnomedicine to that of limited acknowledgment. Doctors no longer scoff at their attempts to integrate ethnomedicine.

Doctors and nurses in Oruro have become more collaborative with ethnomedical practitioners for several reasons: to increase their competitiveness for clientele who come with cultural illnesses, to respond to a growing interest in Andean culture, and to attempt to be more holistic in their therapeutic practices. The workshops in Oruro provided them with knowledge and experiences of ethno-medicine. When ethnomedical practitioners explained what they did and why they did it, some doctors were able to identify with their fellow healers. A wizardly ancient midwife, Doña Matilda, held them spellbound with her wisdom, wit, and midwifery expertise; and in a heated debate over birthing practices, she silenced the doctors with her practical reasons. Doctors and nurses appreciated the ethno-science of Andean medicine after they learned about the topo-graphical-hydraulic model of Kallawaya-Andean ethnophysiology (Bastien 1985). Its logical assumptions and empirical basis erased some stereotypes of it as being based on magic and superstitions.

Clinics with Ethnomedical and Biomedical Practitioners

Clinics with collaborating doctors, nurses, herbalists, diviners, and midwives are a means of coordinating activities between biomedical and ethnomedical practitioners within the community. Since peas-ants in rural communities of Bolivia frequently prefer ethnomedical practitioners, doctors and nurses in clinics in rural areas are often underemployed. Even though the rural health-delivery system has increased threefold in Bolivia, the increment of utilization has been small (*Evaluación* ... 1978). Meanwhile, herbalism and ritual healing are growing in popularity. Integrated clinics draw more patients than do orthodox clinics, in addition to providing a culturally holis-tic approach to illness.

As an early endeavor, members of the ninth Congresso de Medi-cina Natural (November 29, 1979) in La Paz petitioned the Ministry of Health (MPSSP) to establish clinics where doctors and herbalists could collaborate. One was established in La Paz, and others are proposed for Amarete of the Kallawaya region and for Cocapata,

Department of Cochabamba. The latter two were requested by members of their communities. Although, as of 1989, the Cocapata clinic had not started and the status of the Amarete clinic was uncertain, the La Paz clinic has become very successful. It is called *Consultorio SIENS* and is the result of professionally educated Bolivians: doctors, lawyers, and researchers who constitute the Sociedad Boliviana de Medicina Natural (SBMN), La Paz. An ex-Jesuit priest, Jaime Zalles, who practices homeopathic medicine in addition to using sweat baths, directs this clinic, which includes the famous Kallawaya herbalist, Alfonso Ortiz, a medical doctor, a homeopath, and a technician. Patients consult with all practitioners, and therapy is particular to each one. The clinic has also become a center for research on medicinal plants.

One criticism of *Consultorio SIENS* is that it represents more the scientific interests of the middle class than the medical needs of Bolivian peasants. Although I observed several peasants attending this clinic, many patients are middle class Bolivians. More representative of peasants, the SBMN of Oruro was organized by four *qollasiris* (herbalists) from the country, two *naturistas* (nature healers) from the city, two *milluchiris* (masseurs), and two *yatiris* (diviners) and was incorporated on May 24, 1986. These organizers of SBMN sponsored a congress that was to include physicians, and they invited Drs. Oscar Velasco and Betty de Soto to work with them.

Although it is too early to evaluate, many patients have visited this clinic and responded positively to joint therapy. It has been particularly successful in treating *susto*. Initially, doctors objected that the Ministry of Rural Health was paying Velasco and de Soto to work with *curanderos*, but after two years they no longer talked against it and a few doctors refer patients to it. Whenever possible, Dr. Velasco substituted herbal remedies for synthetic drugs. Trained in psychiatry and surgery, he collaborated as a ritual assistant with diviners in therapy for mental illnesses. The following case is an illustration.

Juana was about thirty years old and separated from her husband, who had left her with a small child after she had become disfigured from a burn. While having an epileptic attack, Juana had fallen face first into a fire, leaving her with a badly scarred face. People laughed at her. Her relatives, who were Protestant and who had been told that her troubles were caused by her sinfulness and lack of faith, rejected her. The minister victimized her, which further separated her from the church and her relatives. She retreated to a small community, where she lived with her mother as a recluse,

afraid to go out. The mother called Velasco, who, in several therapeutic sessions, was able to get Juana to look into a mirror and
accept herself. He also reinforced her feelings as a mother and
helped build up her confidence. He gave her medicine to control the
epileptic attacks. In tandem with Velasco's therapy, Juana consulted
a diviner from the clinic, who gathered members of the community
to participate in an all-night ritual. During the ritual, the diviner
symbolically removed the evils attributed to her by the minister, and
the participants joined together in a meal. With Velasco's assistance,
she had plastic surgery and is now a happier person.

Although ideal for physician–indigenous-healer collaboration,
integrated clinics are nevertheless vulnerable to difficulties. One
problem is that sometimes the influence of ethnomedical practitioners in local concerns is subsumed into the bureaucratic and
technocratic influence of the central government. The political
structure of medical care in Bolivia has changed from local oligarchies of administrators, doctors, and nurses to national oligarchies
of the central government's technicians, such as people trained in
sanitation, water projects, immunization, and medicine as well as
technicians from dominant Western countries, be they evangelists,
educators, or community developers. These technicians are not only
displacing the local mestizo oligarchies but also threatening the
influential function of ethnomedical practitioners. Frequently these
technicians forget the role of folk medicine in health care because of
their efforts at consciousness raising of the masses and enforcement
of government policies, project objectives, proselytism, and agrarian
reform (see van den Berghe and Primov 1977:86–87).

Since the Bolivian agrarian reform in 1954, doctors, nurses, auxiliary nurses, and technicians have entered the Bolivian countryside
to improve health. This cadre of educated and progressive young
people slowly took over power from the older, less educated, more
conservative group. Often these rural medical newcomers coalesced
with teachers to form elitist groups of leaders in opposition to the
"backward" traditions of the community. More recently, many doctors, nurses, and auxiliary nurses have become disillusioned, mostly
because of lack of support from the Ministry of Rural Health.
Many have become technocrats trying to control ethnomedical
practitioners.

Another problem of centralization has been that doctors and
nurses are required to make extensive reports to directors in the
Department of Oruro. Rural nurses have to report to as many as
thirteen supervisors in Oruro every two weeks before they are paid.

This information is kept in cardboard boxes in warehouses seldom analyzed for epidemiological data. Instead, outside agencies finance expensive studies by foreigners.

Peasants also realize that their community will receive little or no aid unless they master the paper work and bureaucracy of the health system, and this cannot be done without the assistance of some technician. As a result, local power has shifted from the ethnomedical practitioners to these technicians, whom they have openly opposed. This dissension has stonewalled many health projects and frustrated scores of technicians. Hopefully, if ethnomedical knowledge is incorporated into health planning, its practitioners will not be subservient to biomedical personnel nor succumb to technocratic bureaucracy and its impersonalization.

Summary

Doctors and nurses in Bolivia are collaborating more with ethnomedical practitioners than they did before 1985. There have been concerted efforts to educate biomedical and ethnomedical practitioners on ways that they can collaborate. Workshops in which both types of practitioners discuss how they treat illnesses have proven successful for collaboration in the Department of Oruro. One result has been that doctors and nurses collaborate with ethnomedical practitioners in the treatment of cultural illnesses. Integrated clinics, with both types jointly treating patients, are currently being established in cities and rural areas of Bolivia.

Both types agree that treatment of cultural illnesses is an area where they need to collaborate. Another area not so readily agreed upon is that of immunizations, which is the topic of the next chapter.

8
The Silver Bullet versus the Hexing Thorn

Tetanus—particularly neonatal tetanus—is a terrifying disease found throughout developing countries.* Because neonatal tetanus is so deadly, ethnomedical healers frequently attribute it to pollution, sorcery, and mystical causes. These beliefs can be used to educate people about the preventive powers of vaccinations: the "silver bullet" or syringe can be related to the "hexing thorn" of sorcery. A comparative analysis of cultural perceptions of neonatal tetanus from the slum dwellers of Dhaka, Bangladesh, the Quechua of the Cochabamba Valley, Bolivia, and the Aymaras of the Altiplano and the Tupi-Guarani of Santa Cruz, Bolivia, will show how native concepts can motivate people to participate in tetanus vaccination programs. Collaborative strategies with biomedical and ethnomedical practitioners are needed to educate and convince women to receive the series of tetanus toxoid immunizations to prevent neonatal tetanus.

The Scourge of Lockjaw. Worldwide, tetanus takes the lives of an estimated 441,000 newborns annually (World Health Organization and Expanded Program on Immunization Global Advisory Group 1991). Tetanus, which causes 50 percent of all neonatal deaths and accounts for a quarter of all infant deaths, is second only to measles in its mortality rate. The reporting of neonatal tetanus is extremely incomplete. According to the World Health Organization (1987), the incidence of NNT is only 2 to 8 percent of all reported diseases.

The tetanus bacillus grows anaerobically around agrarian households and frequently enters the bloodstream at birth through the umbilicus when the cord is cut by a contaminated instrument or comes into contact with unclean hands. Symptoms appear from the

* Research for this chapter was supported by the Resources for Child Health Project (REACH) and the United States Agency for International Development (USAID) in Bolivia. Robert Steinglass of REACH was the activity manager; he initiated the project, assisted in the research design, and helped throughout the work. Mike Favin reviewed the chapter and provided useful suggestions. Paul Hartenberger of USAID/BOLIVIA and Wally Chastain of Project Concern provided assistance. Felix Espinosa drove us around Bolivia. Research colleagues Javier Palazuelos and Oscar Velasco greatly assisted in the fieldwork and in the analysis of the data.

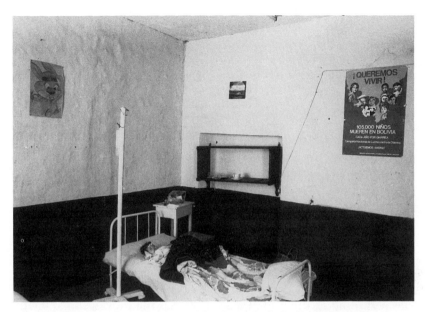

Infant stricken by tetanus in the children's ward of a Bolivian hospital.

third to the tenth day following birth, when the infant is unable to breast-feed. The baby wants to nurse but cannot because of spasms in the jaw muscles. Because these muscles often freeze up, the disease is known by the popular name of "lockjaw" in English. The baby becomes irritable and cries excessively. At first the mother is able to feed the baby by squirting milk into its mouth, but soon this becomes impossible because of the baby's difficulty in swallowing due to spasms of the pharyngeal muscles. Within hours, the body stiffens with convulsive spasms. During these spasms, the arms are flexed at the elbow and held in front of the chest. The fists are tightly clenched, and the toes are dorsiflexed. In severe cases, spasms of the spinal muscles cause the body to arch backwards. Eighty percent of the children thus afflicted die within several days (Galazka and Stroh 1986:1–2).

By vaccinating women with a tetanus toxoid, the deaths could be greatly reduced. In fact, use of tetanus toxoid vaccines could eliminate neonatal tetanus throughout the world. In 1990, however, only 39 percent of pregnant women in the developing world had received at least two tetanus toxoid shots. The objective of WHO's Expanded Program on Immunization is vaccination of all women between fifteen and forty-four years of age, with a schedule of five shots in areas where neonatal tetanus is prevalent. The goal is to have 100 percent coverage by 1995.

Women have resisted this campaign not only because of the pain, effort, and time required but also because they do not see the relevance of immunization since neonatal tetanus is considered a supernatural and traumatic event with psychological, cosmological, and social interpretations. Mothers don't know why five injections are needed nor how these protect their infants from neonatal tetanus. Ethnomedical and biomedical practitioners can facilitate the acceptance of tetanus toxoid vaccinations, and midwives, who do not always practice clean, safe deliveries, can be trained in proper techniques. Until then, neonatal tetanus will continue to strike down infants.

Just as shamanism can be incorporated into the national biomedical health-care system, so too can immunization be incorporated into medical pluralism. However, so long as alternative medical systems exist and specialists within each system have their own theories regarding health and disease, as well as the prevention and curing of diseases, the conflicting perspectives can present obstacles to universal health projects. The Expanded Program of Immunization is a case in point. Started in most countries by 1980, its objective was reducing morbidity and mortality due to diptheria, pertussis, tetanus, poliomyelitis, measles, and tuberculosis by making vaccination services available to all eligible children and pregnant women by 1990. Although this program has been successful in some developing countries, in others it has not met its objectives. Some explanations are lack of properly trained technicians, cultural resistance to and fear of vaccinations, and increased population in rural areas. Ethnomedical practitioners can assist in resolving most of these issues.

Spirit Possession in Bangladesh

Slum dwellers of Dhaka, Bangladesh, refer to tetanus also as *donoshtonkar* and *kichuni* (Blanchet 1989:14–17). They use the English word "tetanus" to refer to convulsions or spasms, sometimes associated with eclampsia (convulsive seizures between the twentieth week of pregnancy and the end of the first week of postpartum). Tetanus is believed to be caused either by the cold, in which case a doctor is called, or by bad air, in which case a fakir healer is called. *Donoshtonkar* designates a disease that is caused when a poison enters the body through a cut or wound. *Kichuni* affects a newborn in the "house of pollution" and is an illness for a fakir healer (Blanchet

1989:13). (Childbirth is culturally associated with uncleanliness, or pollution. Hence, the designation for the birth house.)

The people of Dhaka interpret the symptoms of tetanus according to medical systems of allopathy, homeopathy, and fakir wonderworking. Symptoms become indigenously recognized phenomena according to three cognitive paradigms that have been identified as follows: illness may be given a physiological explanation, it may be attributed to attacks by a spirit, or it may be seen as a punishment for committing a sin.

Traditionally, the symptoms of convulsions, spasms, and rigidity were attributed to possession by spirits (*bhuts*), which mothers recognize as a fatal disease for neonatals. A *bhut* called Chorachuni comes to steal the baby from the house of pollution where mothers are confined for a number of days after the birth. A Chorachuni is a wild jungle spirit who is attracted by the pollution of childbirth. Fighting off this spirit is a lost battle; a mother thinks that her real child has been stolen by the spirit and replaced with a substitute, which is left in her care and which she gives up before it dies (Blanchet 1989:15).

Relatives isolate the mother and the child with tetanus because they believe that a Chorachuni could attack others. The Chorachunis have an appetite for women's eggs, which symbolize sexuality and fertility. They also possess brides and parturient women, killing fetuses in the womb and newborns. After killing a child, a Chorachuni may continue to live with the mother to control her sexuality. Women are not morally blamed when this happens because these spirits are outside the realm of morality and belong to nature (Blanchet 1989:15–16).

A *bhut* enters the mother's and child's bodies through the orifices. Birth leaves the mother dangerously exposed, as does breast-feeding for the infant. A *bhut* prevents infants from nursing by spoiling the mother's milk and causing vomiting and diarrhea. It also strikes infants through bad air or the evil eye. Symptoms of tuberculosis are also associated with a *bhut* in causing a child to lose weight and "dry up" (Blanchet 1989:16).

Many traditional birth attendants use preventive measures to keep evil spirits away from the mother and infant, such as closing off the birth house by magical and material means or by staying awake and burning lamps. Amulets and symbolic objects (pieces of iron, the bones of a sacrificed animal, a broom, an old shoe, a fishing hook and net) are kept near the mother and child (Blanchet 1989:16).

If the symptoms of tetanus are diagnosed as *kichuni* or spirit possession, a fakir is consulted first and a doctor as a second recourse, but only in the cities of Bangladesh, where doctors are gaining some credibility in treating tetanus. Cases of neonatal tetanus admitted to the Dhaka hospital increased fourfold between 1985 and 1988. This figure and the fact that more women are being immunized against tetanus suggest that *kichuni* is slowly becoming a disease for doctors. The people of Bangladesh have been the subject of vaccination campaigns for ten years, with tetanus toxoid receiving the greatest publicity. Before 1980, parents never consulted a doctor for neonatal tetanus; they regarded the doctor's medicine useless to fight the spirit.

As indicated, the slum dwellers of Bangladesh are knowledgeable about the symptoms of tetanus as it affects infants and mothers. Although they traditionally believe the symptoms are caused by spirit possession and are treatable by fakirs, some now recognize that doctors are capable of combating these dreadful symptoms (Blanchet 1989:35). The idea that *kichuni* is caused by spirit possession which can be prevented by protective measures is an apt metaphor for discussing the tetanus toxoid as encoded information that can recognize and resist the tetanus bacteria. Collaboration with fakirs and midwives places these more acceptable healers in an effective position to suggest to pregnant women that they get tetanus toxoid vaccinations as another measure to ward off possessive spirits.

Sorcery and Tetanus among the Quechua of Bolivia

The Department of Cochabamba, Bolivia, has a population of 777,807 people living in 55,631 square kilometers, with a population density of 13.98 people per square kilometer (Muñoz Reyes 1977:2). Here, 141 cases of neonatal tetanus were reported to the Unidad Sanitaria between 1980 and 1986. Forty-six of these cases were fatal. In urban and peri-urban Cochabamba, no symptoms that might suggest neonatal tetanus were identified in a 1991 study by MotherCare Project on reproductive health (Anonymous 1991). Situated in the Yungas area (a lower, humid area from 4,875 to 6,500 ft.), the Chapari region reports the most cases. The District of Aiquile (7,231 ft.) reported seven cases of tetanus in 1987. During Oscar Velasco's and my investigations in Cocapata (7,700 ft.), health personnel reported no incidence of tetanus in this valley. Health personnel of Capinota (8,411 ft.) also claimed that neonatal tetanus did not exist there (Bastien 1988).

Reports from Cocapata and Capinota were questioned in that the health personnel were not clear as to what were the symptoms of neonatal tetanus. Peasants in Cocapata and Capinota raise cows and other livestock associated with tetanus bacilli. Moreover, the parish priest of Capinota said that he had baptized five babies in the last year with symptoms of neonatal tetanus. He reported the same number in outlying rural communities.

This information supported the fact that many cases of neonatal tetanus never arrive at the health posts (*postas sanitarias*) since the affliction is perceived as a bewitchment or *castigo* (punishment) that must be dealt with by ritualists. Because of the stigma and fear attached to this interpretation, peasants do not report neonatal tetanus. Health personnel in the Department of Cochabamba needed to be informed of the symptoms of tetanus so they could collaborate with *curanderos* and priests in its treatment and prevention.

The Quechua frequently refer to tetanus with words that also designate other diseases, such as *tisi onqoy*, which is a combination of *tieso* (rigidity) and *tisis* (tuberculosis) with *onqoy* (sickness); *kharisirisqa*, which refers to acute respiratory infections and diarrhea, attributed to a *kharisiri*, the legendary figure who steals a person's fat; *chujchu* (malaria); *wayra* (Bell's palsy or paralysis); and *arrebato* (fright, or *susto*). No specific name was found for tetanus. Often, Quechua peasants do not recognize rigidity and an infected umbilicus as key diagnostic symptoms. Mothers wrap their infants in wide, woven belts that lessen the possibility of detecting rigidity. They are very concerned, however, when the infant does not breast-feed and has a fever. They cover the umbilicus with raw cotton or rags and are not always aware of its being infected. Often they do not observe the pus excreted from the umbilicus and only report that it is bleeding. Health personnel were instructed to educate women in the mothers' clubs about preventing infections of the umbilicus and recognizing the signs of tetanus in infants as well as—most important—being vaccinated with the tetanus toxoid in order to avoid the disease altogether.

The Quechua attribute many causes to symptoms associated with tetanus. *Wayra* (wind) or *aire* can enter the umbilicus and cause paralysis or *ataques* (convulsions). *Wayra* is also given as the cause of epileptic seizures, heart attacks, Bell's palsy, and polio. This is probably an adaptation of the European humoral theory, which taught that extremes of cold render the blood and muscles immobile. This is also an adaptive strategy to their mountainous region, where there is great fluctuation between night and day temperatures and where icy winds on warm, sweating bodies frequently cause cramps. It is potentially harmful to wash the newborn, which removes protective oils from the skin, subjecting the infant to infection from the cold. *Arrebato (susto)* is another cause of tetanus. The infant loses its *ánimo* because the pregnant mother was nervous, shouted at somebody, lost her temper, or was physically abused. Neither of the two peasants interviewed nor the two auxiliary nurses recognized the relationship between a contaminated umbilicus and neonatal tetanus.

For adults, health personnel attribute tetanus to rusty nails, little aware that the spore is found in dung and on the ground in many courtyards where animals are kept and that the nail is only the means of infection. The probability of people coming into contact with the tetanus spore through injuries to the feet, hands, and legs is high. Finally, they believe that the risus sardonicus, the arched back, and the convulsions are caused by bewitchment. The dramatic nature of tetanus leads peasants to think that its causes lie in the supernatural.

Three classes of cures are employed to treat neonatal tetanus depending on its perceived causes of *susto*, contamination, or bewitchment. *Curanderos* treat *susto* by bathing the infant with herbs, burning *qoa (Satureia boliviana)*, and petitioning the infant's *ánimo* to return. Some perform *santiguadas*, where they incense the child and recite an Our Father and a Hail Mary. They also perform a dispelling ritual, *pichar* (to sweep), to remove "noxious" substances from the infant, which consists of substitution magic: a bundle with undesirable symbols is rubbed on the infant's head, arms, torso, legs, and feet to remove the *chije* (misfortune). This bundle is left at a crossroads for someone else to pick up and harbor the misfortune.

This symbolism can be used to explain how vaccinations work: vaccinations of the tetanus toxoid remove the substances from the woman that cause neonatal tetanus in similar fashion to the *curandero*'s attempts to sweep them from the infant's body, only with the difference that vaccinations protect the infant from getting sick from tetanus in the first place.

As Quechua peasants commonly attribute tetanus to bewitchment and do not consider it a sickness, they bring infants to *curanderos* rather than to the health post. One expert *curandero* from Areque described how he tried to cure an infant with neonatal tetanus. This account provides insights into how Quechuas perceive this disease. Someone envious or hateful of the pregnant mother contracted a *layqa* (witch) to punish the mother by placing a hex on her infant. Infants are more vulnerable than adults, who have more ways of resisting "attacks." The *layqa* made a doll from a stock of black corn, wrapping it with *chumpis* and forming a head. He put cactus spines on one side of the back to cause the baby's body to be arched. He made a frog urinate on the doll and buried the doll near the pregnant woman's house. After the baby boy was born, he appeared to be *asustado*, with his eyes wide open, unable to close them. The mother said that her baby looked at her like a cat without blinking. He opened his hands and could not close them.

The *curandero* was summoned to cure this ten-day-old infant. The mother complained that the infant removed his clothing; she would wrap him up and he would use his strength to undo the wrappings. After the *curandero* threw coca leaves to divine the causes, he told the mother to unwrap the infant because the spell was being cast on a wrapped-up doll. The baby had trouble breathing; his mouth was like that of a fish out of water. He stretched out and retracted from one moment to the next (convulsions). The *curandero* rubbed him with cow grease and alcohol to lower the fever. The infant improved temporarily.

Later in the evening, the parents called the *curandero*, who told them that he was unable to cure the baby and that he should be baptized. They burned *qoa* and prayed because he was like the *sajjra* (devil). The *curandero* washed him with rose water, incense, fox dung, garlic, retama, and alcohol. He feared the strength of the baby. After the bath, the baby improved for a moment, then whimpered softly, his voice rising in a crescendo that ended in the scream of a terrified adult. He raised his head and his eyes protruded as if they were about to pop out. Crying without tears and gasping for air like a fish out of water, he sat up, jerked back, and died. His body was rigid and frozen. Terrified, the *curandero*, the mother, and relatives performed a ritual to protect themselves from the powers of the bewitchment. They sprinkled the blood of white-and-black guinea pigs and sheep around the corners of the house and plaza.

The next day a priest refused to baptize the dead infant, adding to the family's shame and regret. The mother, father, and *curandero* secretly buried the infant in a sacred Quechua burial site, located near the Taquina brewery in Cochabamba.

Several days later, the mother became paralyzed (possibly a hysterical reaction), and the *curandero* cured her with medicinal plants. Because she showed the same symptoms as her baby, he was certain that she was bewitched and recommended that she move from the community. She moved to Oruro and subsequently had six children.

This case history demonstrates that Quechua peasants perceive the symptoms of tetanus within a magical-supernatural framework which not only distresses them but also causes social problems for the family, since the mother is blamed. Neonatal tetanus is perceived more within a social and cosmological context than as a pathological entity. It would be ineffective to try to discount Quechua perceptions, so it is recommended that health personnel be sensitive to these considerations, while at the same time providing alternative therapies and, above all, *stressing preventive immunization*. As mentioned before, one reason why neonatal tetanus cases are not brought to doctors is that the dramatic effect of its symptoms is frequently interpreted as symbolic of witchcraft and devil possession. Moreover, the mother is implicitly and indirectly blamed for this tragedy.

Another insight emerging from this case history is that peasants recognize an infant's vulnerability to the mother's negligence. Blame is implicitly placed on the mother since it is accepted belief that *layqas* frequently attack mothers through their infants because adults have more defenses. Premises of these beliefs can be adapted for vaccination instructions: given that the mother's behavior affects the infant's health, that infants are very vulnerable to attack from outside forces, and that the indirect cause of a symptom in an infant can be traced to the mother (symbolically expressed when the *curandero* threw the coca leaves to ascertain what the mother had done wrong to bring about the bewitchment), then, in a positive fashion, mothers can be instructed that vaccinations are a good way to protect their babies, who are so vulnerable to attacks from foreign things, and themselves from the reproach of the community.

Health workers should not teach germ theory to peasants who have had no exposure to science in school. Neither can peasants living in impoverished areas be expected to create a sterile environment. A more realistic approach would be to suggest a practical and attainable way to *prevent* a disease, such as the tetanus toxoid vaccination.

Claims that the tetanus toxoid prevents the symptoms of tetanus will be understood only in magical-supernatural terms unless peasants are taught the relationship of the microbe to the umbilicus in causing the disease. Although it is not recommended that health educators explain to peasants that the needles of vaccinations protect their babies from the hex-directed thorns of *layqas*, which is unscientific, educators can use this as an analogy to show how vaccinations work. The assumption of witchcraft is that people can cause diseases by negligence and willful acts; so, too, the assumption of immunization is that people can protect themselves and their babies from diseases by freely deciding to be vaccinated five times or with each pregnancy.

Vaccination programs must be conducted as community affairs to utilize a basic Andean concept that health and disease are interrelated to social and cosmological systems. One useful strategy is to invite the *curandero* to participate in the vaccination program by first throwing coca leaves to predict its outcome and then to perform a ritual to make it "complete" or good for the community in a holistic fashion. This can transform someone resistant to vaccinations into a supporter. Moreover, it would also deal with suspicions about the cosmological and social consequences of inserting needles into children and adult women.

Symptom Syndromes among the Aymara of the Altiplano

Doctors and nurses frequently have difficulty diagnosing diseases from symptoms because only 55 percent of the entries in the International Classification of Diseases are scientifically diagnosable, sign and symptom complexes (Janzen 1978:192; World Health Organization 1965). The remaining entries are unrelated signs and symptoms classified somewhat arbitrarily according to body parts and problem focuses. Cultural assumptions, not laboratory assumptions, are the basis for labeling diseases, even in biomedicine.

If a diagnosis reflects cultural assumptions in biomedicine, it does so more in ethnomedicine. The following description of Aymara perceptions of neonatal tetanus illustrates the nebulous connections between the perception of symptoms and tetanus. Aymaras, as well as Quechuas, cluster symptoms that are characteristic of different diseases into culturally defined syndromes. Symptom complexes, such as bewitchment—already discussed above—and *jinchukañu*—discussed below—often include symptoms caused by diseases other than tetanus. Moreover, these symptom complexes are embedded in magical and supernatural symbols.

Health educators are faced with the problem of explaining how vaccinations relate to these culturally defined syndromes. Moreover, it is difficult to separate a disease entity from these symptom complexes, as, for example, to say that some symptoms belong to tetanus and others to tuberculosis. One adaptive strategy is to educate people that they need different vaccinations to take care of multiple symptoms.

Incidence of Tetanus. Tetanus is found less frequently in the Department of Oruro, a part of the Altiplano (12,000 to 13,500 ft.), than in the valleys of Cochabamba and the plains of Santa Cruz. The

Department of Oruro has a population of 310,983 people living in 53,688 square kilometers, with a population density of 5.79 people per square kilometer (Muñoz Reyes 1977:2). Health personnel of the Department of Oruro reported cases of neonatal tetanus in La Joya, Paria, and Totora; all of these communities are above 13,000 feet. These reports dispute recent studies that maintain neonatal tetanus does not exist in the Altiplano, probably because tetanus spores are less frequent in higher altitudes, such as the Altiplano (Marcos de Silveira and Halkyer 1988:1–23). Doctors and nurses from the Ministry of Health cite the Marcos de Silveira and Halkyer study to deemphasize the need for tetanus toxoid vaccinations for Altiplano women.

It seems clear, however, that some tetanus occurs in the Altiplano. Neonatal tetanus is found in communities in the Department of Oruro, but it is reported less frequently than among the Quechua in the valleys of Cochabamba and the Tupi Guarani in the plains of Santa Cruz. Just because neonatal tetanus is seldom reported among the Aymara does not mean it is nonexistent. The epidemiology of neonatal tetanus in Bolivia cannot be determine exclusively by medical records and surveys; it necessitates anthropological investigations together with a surveillance of suspected cases that might not be reported, especially in areas of Bolivia with a presumed high tetanus risk but a low reporting record (Favin et al. 1991). Neonatal tetanus is infrequently reported to the Ministry of Health partly because Aymara peasants do not specify diseases but rather symptom complexes or syndromes, such as *jinchukañu*, which could signify acute respiratory infection, diarrhea, septicemia, meningitis, or neonatal tetanus.

An important factor in transmission is that Aymara women frequently travel to and deliver their babies in lower and more humid areas, where they are at greater risk of contamination from the tetanus spore. This factor warrants tetanus toxoid vaccination for women of the Altiplano. During deliveries, possible sources of contamination are the traditional use of a piece of broken ceramic to cut the umbilical cord, covering it with herbs, and tying it with thread. Midwives place the newborn on a sheepskin—a likely source of tetanus spores—and it is recommended that mothers wash the sheepskin and place it in the sun before it is used for the baby. Men as well as women deliver babies, and frequently their hands are dirty from farm work.

Peasants' Perceptions. As most peasants either do not know the symptoms of neonatal tetanus or do not associate its symptoms with a well-defined disease entity, certain symptoms have priority for Aymara mothers and may mask others. When an Aymara mother, for example, carries on her back a baby that has convulsions and rigidity, is crying excessively, and cannot breast-feed, what concerns her most is the continual crying and the inability to nurse in an infant who previously could nurse. If observed at all, rigidity and convulsions are interpreted as being caused by crying or not feeding. Although constant crying is not a specific symptom of neonatal tetanus, it often indicates to Aymara women that the baby is seriously ill. They do recognize certain types of cries as indicating a grave illness.

Most Aymara peasants do not recognize tetanus as a disease in itself but associate its symptoms with *jinchukañu*, an owl that appears at night and hoots, which sounds like the deep cry of an infant. If the infant cries in return, the owl enters its house as either a cat, insect, or lizard. The owl grasps the baby with its claws. The baby screams, and at this instance its *ajayu* goes from its mouth into the claws of the owl, who flies away. *Ajayu* is frequently translated as "soul" or "spirit" (*ánimo*), but Aymaras perceive it as a vital energizing fluid that is invisible, though important to maintain equilibrium between hot and cold and wet and dry qualities within the body.

Indications of *jinchukañu* are purple marks, supposedly from the owl's claws, found on the baby after death. The symptoms of *jinchukañu* are constant crying, diarrhea, sunken eyes, dry mouth, vomiting, rigidity, fever, and convulsions. This syndrome most frequently refers to acute respiratory infections and diarrhea, but could also apply to bacterial infections of meningitis, septicemia, or neonatal tetanus. Purple spots are physically attributed to lack of oxygen in the infant from respiratory failures, often caused by acute respiratory infections and infrequently by neonatal tetanus in the Altiplano.

Doctors in the Altiplano are unaware that *jinchukañu* is a syndrome that symbolizes several serious diseases as well as magical and mythological realities for Aymara peasants. In many instances the mother is blamed by the community for attacks by *jinchukañu* because she has not guarded the infant. This can be used to motivate her to be vaccinated with the tetanus toxoid as a way to prevent *one* form of *jinchukañu* that results in an infected umbilicus, rigidity, and death.

Curanderos of Zora Zora, Department of Oruro, diagnose *jinchukañu* by giving the infant a drink made from *wilkachapi*, a plant, to see if the infant will vomit, a positive sign of *jinchukañu*. They then place on the infant's stomach a poultice prepared from toasted and crushed yellow pepper seeds. They also have the infant drink a *maté* of *cochinilla*, traditionally used for red dye. *Curanderos* say they can cure some infants of *jinchukañu*, which is probably the case when it is a minor respiratory disease or a mild form of diarrhea. Thus, confusion, mistrust, and even conflict occur when doctors and *curanderos* use the same term but are unwittingly referring to different diseases. For example, doctors investigated a *curandero*'s claim to have cures for cancer and found that he was referring to canker sores.

If the symptoms of *jinchukañu* persist, *curanderos* perform *turka* rituals. A *turka* is the sacrifice of a black male animal (guinea pig, chicken, or pig) in exchange for the *ajayu* of the infant. Blood is sprinkled around the courtyard, and the *curandero* calls the name of the infant so as to recover its *ajayu*. This ritual is commonly called *willancha*. Protestants of Zora Zora have a variation on the *turka* for curing *jinchukañu:* they gather around the infant in prayer and rub its body with the Bible. When this fails, they call a *curandero*. Interestingly, several people began to have doubts about Protestantism when their children died of *jinchukañu*, reasoning that if they had remained Catholic they would have called the *curandero* sooner. Protestants still accept *jinchukañu* as a syndrome even though they do not believe in its magical causes. Nevertheless, *jinchukañu* also constitutes a defense mechanism of ethnomedicine for *curanderos* because it puts into serious conflict those peasants who have abandoned the rituals of *curanderos* for the Bible to fend off the owl.

These data show that *jinchukañu* is a syndrome of deadly diseases for infants, but which is perceived by Aymara peasants within a religious-mythological framework where ritual is the culturally preferred treatment. It is difficult to convince them otherwise, because this belief is culturally validated and operates with different epistemological criteria than those of biomedicine. However, health workers can adapt medical therapies for infants with *jinchukañu* by consulting with *curanderos* and offering to assist them in the curing and prevention of it. One way to do this is to have the *curanderos* perform a *turka* ritual the night before the women are vaccinated. According to Dr. Edgar Francken, medical supervisor in this region, nurses and community health workers in Culta and Zora Zora of the Curahuara de Carangas Province, Bolivia, have collaborated with *curanderos* and have a 100 percent vaccination rate for children. They have recently begun tetanus toxoid vaccinations for women.

One concept that can be used to promote vaccinations is to remind Aymaras how in past times getting vaccinated eliminated smallpox. They still recount how some peasants vaccinated themselves with pus from another's sores. Also recalled was a nurse explaining how *alfombrillo*, measles, had been stopped in a community where he had vaccinated all the children, but how in another community they had refused and many children had died.

Health workers can talk about *jinchukañu* as a syndrome that can be caused by several diseases, respiratory infections, diarrhea, meningitis, septicemia, polio, and tetanus, some of which can be prevented by vaccinations. To adopt a holistic approach, the health-care workers can say that they will prevent *jinchukañu* and that mothers, children, community health workers, nurses, midwives, and *curanderos* will all cooperate in the endeavor. Mothers must be vaccinated multiple times with the tetanus toxoid, and children three times against diphtheria, pertussis, and tetanus and once against measles and tuberculosis. Children should also receive drops on three occasions to prevent polio. Community health workers are needed to explain the complex interrelationship of *jinchukañu* to vaccinations, and *curanderos* can perform rituals to prevent *jinchukañu* and to participate in the campaign against childhood diseases. They also need to prevent diarrhea and administer oral rehydration therapy to babies who have it. Midwives need to provide clean standards for the delivery of babies. Nurses need to explain the diseases prevented by vaccinations and their reactions. Ironically, the fact that Aymaras perceive diseases within such a holistic perspective as *jinchukañu* impedes health personnel from adopting a simplistic and mechanistic approach to eliminating tetanus as well as other diseases, some of which are intimately linked to economic, social, and cultural factors.

Culture-Specific Approaches. Underlying themes useful for educators are that *jinchukañu* can symbolize something very aggressive against the infant, can indicate the seriousness of the symptoms, and can imply that the parents are responsible for neglecting the child. These themes can easily be transferred to the dangers of the tetanus microbe in attacking the infant, the devastating symptoms of neonatal tetanus, and the irresponsibility of the mother not to have been vaccinated.

Doctors and nurses need to examine carefully infants with *jinchukañu* to ascertain from this syndrome which ones correspond to modern pathology. Health personnel contend that neonatal tetanus is not recognized in the Altiplano, but if they question peasants about *jinchukañu* they will find it in a minority of these cases.

A culturally appropriate symbol for the vaccination card would be an image of the *Virgen de Copacabana,* which represents fertility, protection, motherhood, Mother Earth *(Pachamama),* and earth. The color of the cards could be bright pink, a favorite color of Aymara women. The card must be large, with several illustrations symbolizing protection, such as a mother guarding her infant, a dog protecting some lambs, and a cat chasing away rodents. The term *jinchukañu* should not be used on the card because it may not be universally understood by Aymaras of the Altiplano.

Miasma, Tetanus, and the Tupi-Guarani of Santa Cruz, Bolivia

The following description of neonatal tetanus among the Tupi-Guarani, Department of Santa Cruz, Bolivia, illustrates problems health educators confront when people hold on to older theories of contagion, such as miasma. Miasma refers to a foul emanation or odor from the earth thought to cause diseases endemic to the region. Until the cholera epidemic in England early in the nineteenth century, doctors explained miasma as the cause of epidemics. The term "malaria," *mal aire,* is a metaphor for miasma. When ethnomedical systems follow a different medical theory, then health educators need to understand this logic and devise explanations to deal with it. Even today, many people believe that colds are caused by drafts of cold air and not viruses, which derives from the Hippocratic/Galenic humoral theory of the balance between the hot and the cold necessary for health.

The peasants of Santa Cruz believe that tetanus is caused not by microbes, but by smells, vapors, and wind. Neonatal tetanus is called *pasmo de ombligo,* and is attributed to a cold blast of air or wind *(wayra)* chilling the baby or mother, resulting in paralysis or *ataques* (convulsions). Thus, doctors must realize that these peasants do not consider contamination and lack of hygiene, especially in regard to birth practices (cutting and tying of the umbilical cord), as causes of tetanus.

Incidence of Tetanus. Neonatal tetanus is endemic in the Department of Santa Cruz, with a population of 712,407 people in an area of 370,621 square kilometers and a density of 1.92 per square kilometer (Muñoz Reyes 1977:2). Neonatal tetanus is commonly found in Districts I and II (from sea level to 2,000 ft.) of the department. District I reported thirty-four cases from January to June 1988 out of a pop-

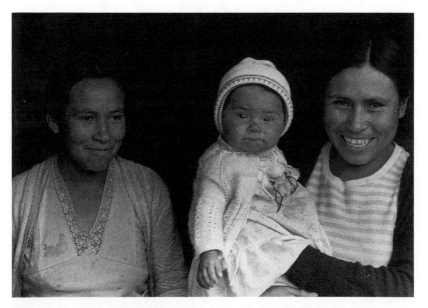

Tupi-Guarani women and child from Department of Santa Cruz. They believe
tetanus is caused by smells, vapors, and wind.

ulation of 119,960 people, which gives an annual reported neonatal
tetanus mortality rate of 13.2 per 1000 live births. District II
reported sixty-seven cases in 1985, eighty-one in 1986, and sixty-five
in 1987, with the large communities of Montero recording ninety-
one, Mineros twenty-four, and Sagrado Corazon twenty-nine cases
over this three-year period (Ayala Benitez and Torrico Espinoza
1988). In Jorochito, a community outside of Santa Cruz, the incidence of neonatal tetanus nearly doubled from seven in 1983 to
thirteen in 1987.

In the Hospital de Niños, Montero, 10 to 15 percent of the
patients were sick from neonatal tetanus (Montaño Cuéllar 1985;
Torrico Espinoza 1987). Admitted were five- to ten-day-old infants
weighing over three kilos. Out of a total of 208 cases (1980–86), 130
(62.5 percent) were boys and 78 (37.7 percent) were girls. Most had
been delivered by the mother's own mother, other relatives, or midwives and were from rural areas. Prior to being hospitalized, the
majority of infants had been treated by family members and *curanderos*. Doctors reported a relatively high success rate in treatment,
compared to other parts of the world, with 146 (70 percent) of the
infants recovering and 62 dying. This very low fatality rate raises
some doubt as to the reliability of these doctors' diagnoses and sug-

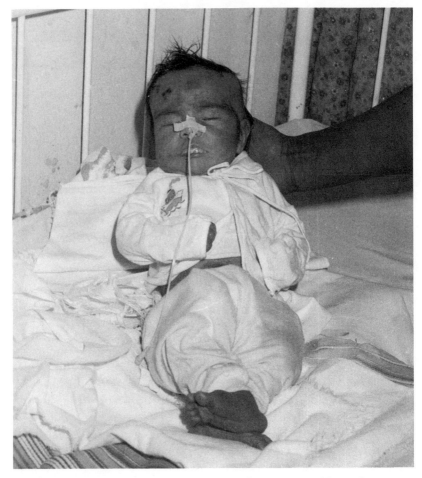

Infant dying of neonatal tetanus in Montero, Department of Santa Cruz.

gests that the infants recovered from other illnesses (R. Steinglass, pers. com. 1988).

The fact that the majority of neonatal cases in Montero were babies delivered by midwives and relatives indicates the lack of hygiene as a probable cause. They cut the umbilical cord with knives, scissors, broken glass or ceramic pieces, rocks, human hair, and corn leaves. They tie it with string or hair and put dandelion and *lengua de buey* herbs on it. These unsterilized items frequently come into contact with tetanus bacilli. One possible explanation for why more boys than girls contact neonatal tetanus in Montero is that TBAs leave a longer section of the umbilical cord for the boy that is more likely to become infected. Birth attendants often do not wash themselves or the baby because they fear contamination by cold air, and they often wrap the baby with unwashed cloths.

As discussed in chapter 6, it is difficult to reeducate midwives since they follow indigenous practices. Few understand germ theory, and almost all use available materials in their practice. In Vallegrande, for instance, a mother on a journey delivered her own baby by cutting the umbilical cord with two stones, and the infant died of tetanus. At meetings of mothers' clubs, health personnel can assist expecting mothers to prepare birth delivery kits containing a sealed razor blade, sterilized cotton and thread, and alcohol. Midwives and mothers must be discouraged from using medicinal plants to dress the umbilical cord.

Etiology and Treatment. Tupi-Guarani peasants do not associate the infected umbilicus with the cause of neonatal tetanus; they cluster this symptom into a *pasmo* syndrome, which includes symptoms indicative of emanations from the environment. They perceive *pasmo de ombligo* either as a drying up or a congealing of the body brought about by toxic odors or cold winds, which cause an imbalance of vital fluids. A deeper look at the word *pasmo,* however, reveals its etiology. *Pasmos* are often associated with elements of the universe, such as *pasmo de la luna, pasmo del rayo, pasmo del sol,* and *pasmo del sur. Pasmos* are believed to be caused, for example, when the mother exposes her infant to different climatic elements. *Pasmo del rayo* is caused by the pregnant mother being exposed to lightning, and leads to the child having epileptic seizures. *Pasmo del sol* is over-exposure of the infant to the sun, which results in fever, and *pasmo de sereno* is produced by humid nights and results in respiratory diseases. The Tupi-Guarani classify *pasmos* into those that are *caliente* (hot) and those that are *frios* (cold), depending on whether the infant is sweating or rigid.

From the above uses of *pasmo,* one can interpret *pasmo de ombligo* to mean that some emanation from the earth has passed from the mother through the umbilical cord to the child. For example, one cause of *pasmo de ombligo* is if the pregnant mother walks past putrid matter, such as a cemetery or a dead dog. It is the *odor* that causes the disease.

Native practitioners have no specific treatments for tetanus, per se, but many for *pasmo de ombligo.* They bathe the infant with herbs and ashes of worn clothes and soles of shoes. Another treatment is to place the baby in the intestinal cavity of a slaughtered cow, symbolizing its rebirth. They also burn oils from cow's hooves and resin of the *cuti* tree around the infant. They place plasters of *puchon* oil mixed with scrapings of *wayacan* and, in other instances, of *cutuqui* on the infected umbilicus. These herbal remedies treat the symptoms: they lower the fever, control secretions from the umbilicus, increase blood pressure, and relieve congestion. This also supports the conclusion that sicknesses other than tetanus are included in *pasmo de ombligo*, some of which *curanderos* are able to cure.

Health personnel could educate *curanderos* that an infected umbilicus possibly indicates neonatal tetanus, which can be prevented by tetanus toxoid vaccinations. *Curanderos* should be invited to participate in vaccination campaigns and given credit for preventing this disease.

Mothers bring infants with neonatal tetanus to ritualists. Although a variety of rituals can be found throughout the Department of Santa Cruz, a fairly typical pattern is to have ritualists perform *la santiguada* and *saraqoa* for *pasmo de ombligo*. *Santiguadores* incense the child and then pray a *Padre Nuestro* (Our Father) and an *Ave Maria* over the child. They call this *"una vencida,"* "conquering the other force." Meanwhile, relatives call the name of the child to recover its *ánimo* or *ajayu*. *Saraqoa* is a ritual of Andean origin, probably introduced by Aymara and Quechua migrants. Ritualists sacrifice a sheep, eat it in a communal meal, and bury its bones at a crossroads. They *pichan* (sweep) the body of the infant with these bones to remove the substance causing the sickness.

When *pasmo de ombligo* is tetanus, these rituals are unsuccessful and the baby is brought to the priest for baptism. For most peasants throughout Bolivia, baptism is more important than hospitalization in cases of gravely ill neonates because they fear that unbaptized babies become *moros* (infidel Moors) or *demonios* (devils) who will plague their communities with hail, drought, floods, and frosts. Priests are in a position to arrange for collaborative treatment of *pasmo de ombligo* by doctors. The Episcopal Conference of Bishops of the Catholic Church could issue a pastoral letter advising married women to receive the tetanus toxoid and instructing all priests to refer cases of seriously ill infants brought for baptism to doctors.

Culture-Specific Approaches. Doctors and nurses might try these culture-specific messages and approaches for tetanus toxoid vaccinations among the Tupi-Guarani:

1. Tetanus is a deadly form of *pasmo de ombligo* that causes rigidity,

convulsions, and death in infants. Tetanus is an invisible living organism found in the soil. This organism frequently sticks to the hands and instruments of the person performing the home delivery and enters the umbilicus of the baby. The baby becomes very sick with a rigid mouth, arched back, convulsions, and often fever. The baby usually dies from this form of *pasmo de ombligo.*

2. Mothers cry when their babies die because they love them so. Their children bring them happiness, but not when they die from *pasmo de ombligo.* One type of *pasmo de ombligo,* tetanus, can be prevented from killing infants. Mothers can protect their babies from tetanus by receiving the protective fluids of tetanus toxoid injections. These valuable fluids pass from the injection into the mother and through the umbilical cords to their babies. These fluids, called tetanus toxoid, protect the babies for a while from the rigid form of *pasmo de imbligo.* Soon after birth, babies must receive their own protective fluids by being vaccinated for diphtheria, pertussis, and tetanus.

This message can be printed on tetanus toxoid vaccination cards given to women. Explanations that need to be included are: women from menarche to menopause need to be vaccinated because this is the childbearing age and many of their children die from neonatal tetanus; multiple doses are necessary so that women are continually protected; reactions are slight fevers and headaches, for which aspirins can be taken; and what the schedule is for the vaccinations. Instead of printing five spaces to be marked each time the woman is vaccinated, it is better to print the meaning of each inoculation. For example, with the third dose: during the next five years, a mother will protect her newborn infants from *pasmo de ombligo* (tetanus). Care must be taken not to confuse the duration of the mother's protection with that of the infant. A culturally appropriate symbol to mark the vaccinations would be a cross, which contains several meanings (Jesus, protection, earth, and sky), and suggests a syringe. The above suggestions need to be field-tested before adoption.

Cross-Cultural Similarities

The four ethnographic descriptions of the incidence and treatment of neonatal tetanus illustrate some important aspects regarding the collaboration between bio- and ethnomedicine. The four cultural areas share the similarity that neonatal tetanus is perceived within a magical and biological framework that involves alternative healing systems and healers. They employ cognitive paradigms of alternative systems, such as allopathy, homeopathy, home cures, and elaborate cosmological systems embedded in ritual. Healers are doctors, nurses, vaccinators, fakirs, priests, *curanderos,* shamans, midwives, and herbalists.

Another common characteristic is that peoples from the four cultural areas had diffuse knowledge about the symptoms of neonatal tetanus and associated specific symptoms of tetanus with a variety of other illnesses. The people of Bangladesh associated tetanus with eclampsia, Bell's palsy, and poisoning. The Quechua confused it with epileptic seizures, Bell's palsy, and polio, and the Aymara with septicemia, acute respiratory infections, and meningitis. The Tupi-Guarani confused it with a score of illnesses related to emanations from the earth. Tetanus is not a clearly marked target for these people.

Examples have been given to suggest how doctors and nurses can educate peoples of these cultures concerning neonatal tetanus and tetanus toxoid vaccinations. That vaccinations help mothers and their infants respond to tetanus must be communicated using accurate convergent concepts understandable to members of the culture. Health educators need to be careful to focus on the specific symptoms of tetanus identified by each culture as being preventable by tetanus toxoid vaccinations. This is to avoid misunderstandings by the people that all the symptoms of the culturally defined syndromes will be prevented by tetanus toxoid vaccinations. Health educators can emphasize that various types of vaccinations are needed to prevent some of the symptoms of these culturally defined illnesses.

The lesson for biomedical practitioners is that people have been resistant to vaccination campaigns because of misinformation, authoritarian treatment, and lack of cross-cultural communication skills on the part of vaccinators. A knowledge of how people understand neonatal tetanus can better enable biomedical personnel to be more holistic in preventive medicine.

Avoiding Failure in Communicating: Sharing Information Cross-Culturally

The task of universal immunization programs calls for enormous efforts in planning, synchronization, and management; logistics are only a part of the overall job. The failure of the Expanded Program of Immunization has been that it has not persuaded village people to give injections and drops to healthy infants and women. Generally speaking, people use biomedicine to be cured, and if they are healthy, they avoid it. "Why should healthy people receive injections?" they ask. And if the health worker replies that the mother should receive tetanus toxoid vaccinations so that the child receives her immunity and does not die of neonatal tetanus, then they reply that children do not die of tetanus, they die from *pasmo de ombligo, jinchukañu,* or bewitchment. Healthy women and children do not understand why they must be painfully vaccinated and suffer reactions.

Doctors and nurses need to educate people on preventive medicine, employing concepts of allopathic and homeopathic medicine from both scientific and cultural perspectives. Not only are the theoretical bases of allopathic and homeopathic medicines different but also allopathic medicine itself can appear to be somewhat contradictory. The allopathic medicine that doctors and nurses employ to cure disease induces a pathologic reaction antagonistic to the disease being treated. Immunizations, however, are similar to homeopathic medicine in that small substances of a disease similar to the one to be prevented are injected into the person to activate immunities and prevent the more dreaded disease. Excluding immunizations, homeopathic medicine has little acceptance by doctors and nurses who are not trained to educate people in its concepts.

As illustrated in the case studies, ethnomedical systems frequently employ preventive and homeopathic medicines. Slum dwellers in Bangladesh, for example, prevent illnesses by amulets, appropriate foods, baths, blessings of elders, ritual purity, and doing one's duty (Blanchet 1989:27). Although these practices assume that illnesses are caused by unappeased spirits, violations of the cosmic order, breaking a taboo, or disrupting the social order, the idea is that something can be done to prevent illnesses. Even though it is difficult to educate peasant people about vaccinations, they understand prophylactic amulets and rituals. Some groups pay homage to the deities of sicknesses. Shamans are frequently persons who have survived lethal diseases and claim the skill to cure them as a consequence. Aymara peasants in the Altiplano, however, took pus from festulated smallpox sores of an infected person and vaccinated themselves to prevent this deadly disease. In short, ethnomedical systems include the notion of prevention, be it preventing ghosts from inflicting illnesses by prophylactic sorcery or using preventive measures that are the equivalent of biomedical immunization.

One unfortunate practice has been that doctors and nurses frequently administer vaccinations without explanation. In the style of a past colonial epoch, they order the "natives" to line up and get shot by the "silver bullet." As one health planner from India said, "The beauty of vaccination programs is that they require little from the community beyond lining up and holding out their arm at the proper time. . . . It matters little whether a soldier understands the principles of how the rifle works as long as he knows how to aim, load, and shoot. It is the same with vaccinations" (Nichter 1990:197). The military model uses the image of weapons for vaccinations, which, like allopathic medicine, are quick fixes to destroy the enemy.

In contrast, Nichter (1990) suggests a shared-information model for immunization that may bring significant positive results: Doctors and nurses explain vaccinations as encoded information that enters the body through the needle and provides the body an opportunity to recognize danger. They illustrate how vaccines help the body recognize and respond to antigens as producers of harmful toxins or agents wanting to exploit the cells. Doctors can then describe what the various antigens are and what vaccines are needed to respond to them. Health educators can also teach other measures to recognize and respond to these antigens, such as using a microscope to show people that the tetanus bacteria is found on unsterilized knives used to cut umbilical cords, which causes neonatal tetanus, and that they can prevent this by sterilizing the knife.

Doctors must adapt the information model of immunization to peoples' conceptions, etiologies, and treatment of immunofacient diseases. In short, a cross-culturally sensitive information model must be implemented to change widespread resistance to vaccinations throughout the world. The cases discussed in this chapter illustrate this need.

Ethnomedical practitioners can assist greatly in immunization programs, as illustrated in Oruro, Bolivia, in 1987 to 1988. The organization of ethnomedical curers (SOBOMETRA) and La Unidad Sanitaria (Ministry of Health) cooperated in a program of immunizations and oral rehydration therapy. Ethnomedical practitioners administered certain immunizations and helped unite people at vaccination centers. Some ethnomedical practioners fully supported this activity, while others, especially *naturistas* (nature healers), criticized it for being affected and tokenism. The ethnomedical practitioners who were supportive said that it was an excellent way to prevent diseases and deaths in children (Oscar Velasco, pers. com. 1988). In Santa Cruz, traditional birth attendants have received training in preventive measures over the last two years, and are now giving tetanus toxoid injections (Favin et al. 1991).

9
Conclusions

The most evident medical trend of the twentieth century has been biomedicine—multinational pharmaceutical businesses, globalized government support, scientific universality, homogenized techniques, and by-the-book doctors. Amid this bustling bigness, political control, and homogenization is heard the persistent cry of tradition, individuality, and community out of a sense that comforting certainties of culture are being stripped away. Patients face alone the cold, clinical reality of physicians and operating rooms. Where once people believed that creators, spirits, and ancestors intervened to strike and heal, now they despairingly realize that they are at the mercy of science and doctors. Their gods have been replaced by the "major deities" or MDs of the medical profession.

If one can predict medical trends of the next century, then the movement toward consolidation and homogenization focused around biomedicine will be modified by incorporation of alternative medical systems into health care. This prediction has shaped the chapters in this book.

"Why can't people accept the fact that illnesses are biological facts and best treated by biomedical technicians?" is the standard scientific objection to the supposedly "quacky" practices of ethnomedical healers. When illness is stripped from the eternal to the minimal, then doctors are right. But the fact is that people die of incurable diseases, and illness shakes the very fiber of people's reality. Illnesses are not only natural but also cultural entities, demanding the best of religious, psychosocial, and cosmological systems to support.

The Selling of the Shaman

At a time when doctors are trying to replace ethnomedical therapies with biomedical practices in developing countries, patients in the developed world are rediscovering ethnomedical healing. A very striking example is that members of the "New Age movement" and many others have adopted shamanism (Joralemon 1990). Mostly middle-class patients attend "Native American Healing Vacation Workshops" at the Joy Lake Mountain Seminar Center in Reno to be

215

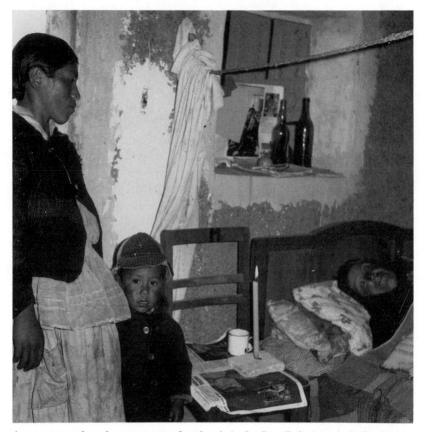

Aymara grandmother prepares for death in La Paz. Religious beliefs play an important role in the management of illness and death; ritualists assist with this transition.

cured or trained in "shamanic trance and lucid dreaming" at the Transformative Art Institute. Ethnologist of Jivaro shamans, Michael Harner offers training in "shamanic counseling" at the Foundation for Shamanic Studies in Norfolk, Connecticut. The popularity of "neo-shamanism" is very high in West Germany, the most industrialized country in the world (Doore 1988). Witchcraft is also popular in West Germany.

New Agers. Shamans have changed and become internationally popular to meet the commercial needs of tourist agencies and the spiritual/medical needs of "New Agers." Tony Agpasa is an internationally known psychic healer and *espiritista* in the Philippines, who treats patients from the United States and elsewhere.

Otherworld Tours, Inc., and the Four Winds Foundation lead tours with Eduardo Calderón to Peru "to return to the Pachamama, Mother Earth" and "meet the Beings of Light still present at ancient initiatory and ceremonial sites" (Joralemon 1990:108). Calderón is a Peruvian north coast shaman made famous by Doug Sharon's book *Wizard of the Four Winds*, his movie *Eduardo the Healer*, and a twelve-part TV series, *Healing States: Doorways to the Spirit World*, directed by Alberto Villoldo. Calderón is able to shift from Peruvian idioms of indigenous patients' distress to those of foreigners on his tour. In a ritual with Peruvians and tourists present, he explains sickness in terms of *daño* (sorcery-induced "harm") to the natives and as having "a good third eye" to the tourists. On these tours, he changes traditional rituals to suit the cultural community of the tourists. He provides guidelines that are congruent with the beliefs of the patients.

One stop on the curing tour takes place at a lagoon where Calderón tells tourists that they are entering into the spirit world. Group members strip naked, throw personal objects into the water, and then line up to be rubbed with a sword by Calderón. He tells them that he is cutting away connections to the past so that they can be born again as shamans. He spins the participants in one direction and then in the other, and sends them to roll in the mud (Joralemon 1990:109). Of this, he says, "After we spin out of our old selves we roll in the earth, born this time not of woman but Mother Earth herself." He then blows sacred herbs on the tour members. Villoldo filmed this curing tour, and informs the audience that "many medicine men believe that the time has come to share their knowledge with the white man, that the new shaman, the new caretakers and healers of the earth must come from the West" (Joralemon 1990:109).

From the wings of the clinics came scoffs at such outlandish practices, interpreted as similar to TV evangelists duping the "yuppie" middle class and sick people in search of a cure. And the whole operation didn't seem correct, at least not very hygienic unless you believe in mud baths. However, while that may be true (or not), it is also clear that these "tourists" are looking for alternative medical systems which include spiritual, earthly, cosmological, and even feminine dimensions.

Conjunctures of Cultures. The irony is that people from industrialized countries are traveling to developing countries to learn about ethnomedicine, and people from developing countries are traveling to industrialized countries to learn about biomedicine. Thus, there exists the rich possibility of dialogues between people of different cultures to examine alternative medical systems.

As discussed, there are many ways that practitioners of biomedicine and of ethnomedicine can collaborate. This collaboration is necessary to modify extremes of each type of practitioner. With their scientific orientation, doctors can help shamans select techniques healthy to the patient. With their sociocultural orientation, ethnomedical practitioners can help doctors be more culturally sensitive. As in the case of Calderón and the tourists, the bizarre approach is good business, but it is not necessarily good healing. As for the doctors, biomedical healing is even more profitable as a business, but it is not personally fulfilling for many patients.

Missed Opportunities. If biomedical personnel do not integrate their work with that of ethnomedical practitioners, many opportunities will be missed to provide public health measures to a lot of people. Many patients do not go to clinics and hospitals, so they are not available for immunizations. They do, however, visit herbalists and midwives who, if they are integrated into public health programs, can either immunize or instruct them to be immunized. In Haiti, as an example, midwives refuse to deliver a baby unless the mother has been vaccinated because they don't want to be blamed if the infant dies of neonatal tetanus (Gretchen Berggren, pers. com. 1990).

The collaboration of doctors and ethnomedical practitioners is necessary to help patients and their ethnomedical practioners distinguish practices that are worthwhile from those that are not. Examples throughout this book clearly demonstrate that some indigenous cures are worthwhile because they are efficacious, some are worthwhile because they are embedded in sociocultural relations, and some are not worthwhile. Doctors need to assist ethnomedical practitioners and patients in distinguishing the latter from the former two—and in a way that is collaborative, not authoritative.

Biomedical Healers and Collaboration

Biomedical personnel present the biggest obstacle to pluralistic medical systems. Their control of health care is deeply rooted in economic, political, and discursive power (Foucault 1975; Illich 1976; Starr 1982). The majority of doctors scarcely recognize or value therapeutic practices of alternative medical systems. Moreover, they make little effort in dealing with the cultural, social, and psychological aspects of illnesses. They are encapsulated within a biomedical paradigm which assumes that science dictates medical policy. This has become the epistemology of their tightly controlled and wealthy medical system.

Nonetheless, chapters in this book discuss ways in which doctors and nurses in Bolivia and other parts of the world can collaborate with ethnomedical practitioners. This collaboration is effective when doctors recognize, respect, and reward ethnomedical practitioners and train them to record patients' medical history and to make referrals.

Recognition. Biomedical practitioners need to recognize the legitimacy of ethnomedical healers. Recognition has come a long way from the days when ethnomedical practitioners were persecuted and disparaged by government officials and doctors who believed that indigenous practitioners were frauds. In many countries, such as Bolivia, laws were passed in the 1930s and 1940s making the practice of these healers illegal, so they practiced covertly, begetting even less recognition.

Fortunately, this suppression has decreased, although ethnomedical practitioners are still wary. An increasing number of biomedical personnel are accepting of ethnomedical practitioners for a number of reasons. Medical anthropologists and ethnoscientists have helped people understand how alternative therapy works. Ethnomedical practitioners contribute to medicine with medicinal plants, psychosocial healing, birth deliveries, and preventive medicine. And the laws were reversed after the Bolivian Agrarian Reform in 1954. Because of lingering memories of suppression, doctors must take the initiative to collaborate by first building trust between them and ethnomedical practitioners.

Recognition implies that doctors and nurses study the practices of ethnomedical practitioners. Once doctors and nurses are knowledgeable about these practices, they have some criteria for evaluating them and for determining how they can collaborate with ethnomedical practitioners. Doctors can learn indirectly by reading ethnographic studies of the practices of healers, now available for most cultural areas of the world, but they would benefit far more by inviting these healers to demonstrate their curing techniques. Ethnomedical healers welcome the opportunity to be recognized by doctors and nurses. In return, doctors and nurses could invite ethnomedical healers to observe treatment of patients in the clinic or surgery room of the hospital. Rarely, if ever, has a midwife been invited to deliver a baby in the delivery room of a hospital. In fact, instructions for midwives are conducted outside of delivery rooms because they are not allowed into them.

Doctors and nurses frequently have trouble recognizing which ethnomedical healers are most influential in the community. This has been a persistent problem in the training of midwives. The midwives who are trained are often young, literate women, sent by the men of the village for political reasons, and are infrequently called upon to deliver babies. An effective way to find out who are the popular healers is to ask the mothers of the village who delivered their babies or to ask patients in a clinic which healers they have consulted. Frequently, doctors recognize only ethnomedical healers peripheral to the peasant community because they are most like them (speaking European languages, literate, and understanding some biomedicine). Because these healers are marginal to the community, they are often disliked by more influential healers. By collaborating only with them, doctors further distance themselves from the influential healers of the community.

Recognition also implies that doctors include healers in planning and implementing health programs. Ethnomedical healers are essential for planning in that they provide encapsulated information in a ritual or therapeutic session on the values, perceptions and attitudes of the clients. The knowledge, attitude, and practices (KAP) of clients has become an integral part of public health work within this decade. KAP requires that doctors be sensitive to the clients' culture so they can communicate effectively. As illustrated throughout this book, many ethnomedical healers are experts on this. Far better than anthropologists, healers can help health workers integrate KAP into their programs, but anthropologists are essential to facilitate this process.

Regarding implementation, ethnomedical practitioners are usually adept at connecting culturally coded messages with healing practices. Doctors, however, frequently stick to the technical aspects of medicine without regard for imagery, feelings, and motivation. Doctors could utilize healers in providing images, rituals, and symbols for public health measures. As shown in chapter 8, one shaman suggested that because Quechuas of Cochabamba perceive neonatal tetanus as being caused by a needle driven into a doll, this image can be used to explain that the vaccination syringe is another needle protecting the mother and child against this danger of tetanus. Where biomedical personnel have failed is in the use of imaginative ways to communicate biomedical technology to people; consequently, people have not been motivated to accept these innovations.

As already mentioned, doctors and nurses need to recognize the many opportunities that ethnomedical healers provide for the implementation of health programs: midwives for tetanus toxoid vaccinations of mothers and other vaccines for children, herbalists for family planning, shamans for education on nutrition, and community health workers for record keeping. Because ethnomedical healers are found in many communities, they provide additional personnel to employ for health programs. Without their assistance, doctors and nurses, already in short supply, will be unable to accomplish rural coverage for health programs. Not to recognize the role of ethnomedical healers in the implementation of health programs is a frequent and tragic "missed opportunity."

Respect. Respect implies that doctors treat ethnomedical practitioners with trust, dignity, and equality as colleagues. Doctors often believe that they are the exclusive and most effective healers and that all other healers are charlatans. This myopic view of health has led to a monopolistic control of medicine by biomedical personnel. Ethnomedical healers are then evaluated according to biomedical standards, which is like playing basketball on a football field. According to these standards, ethnomedical practitioners are denied respect and lose legitimacy.

The argument presented in this book is that there are many effects of alternative therapies little considered in biomedicine, such as psychological, spiritual, social, cultural, and environmental ones. Case studies exemplified some effects that ethnomedical healers have on the total well-being of the person. Disregard for all healing practices outside the biomedical tradition ignores time-tested methods people have used to adapt to their environment with available resources and personnel. Consider how the shaman in Qaqachaka helped Inez adjust to village life, or how Kallawaya herbalists used plants of tropical and mountain zones to cure ailments.

Respect includes autonomy. With reason, ethnomedical healers fear that if they are incorporated into the dominant medical system they will be controlled by doctors, lose flexibility and patients, and be absorbed into the biomedical system. This fear can only be overcome by a respect that permits alternative healers to practice their art as they have learned and adapted it to the needs of the people. One way to promote equality and autonomy is to have a director of indigenous medicine within the Ministry of Health. A successful example of this was presented in chapter 7 for Bolivia. The Ministry of Health in the Department of Oruro first named Dr. Oscar

Velasco, M.D., and later Dr. Betty de Soto, M.D., as directors of eth-nomedical medicine for this region. Their role was to acknowledge the benefits of ethnomedicine, to suggest avenues of collaboration, and to guarantee the autonomy of ethnomedical practitioners. Because Velasco and de Soto were knowledgeable about ethnomedi-cine and respected the autonomy of indigenous healers, they were able to help other doctors do the same. Another measure to assure autonomy is for ethnomedical healers to form associations indepen-dent of doctors, as will be discussed later.

Doctors should respect the beliefs of ethnomedical practitioners so long as they are not harmful to the patient's health. If beliefs are harmful, doctors can teach healers in a sensitive manner how to replace these beliefs. Doctors have published lists of harmful prac-tices without regard for the feelings of alternative practitioners, resulting in the incrimination of healers as being harmful to patients. Respect implies that doctors recognize the cultural context of harmful practices and intelligently replace them with others that are not. If doctors do this, ethnomedical practitioners will be more receptive to these changes because they can understand the harm and will know how to fix it without their practice being threatened.

Moreover, biomedical personnel need to respect the part that magic, ritual, and theatrics play in healing: they can no longer write these culturally oriented therapies off as quackery. Biomedical per-sonnel know little about the role of religion in healing. This is an area where ethnomedical healers can teach doctors a great deal.

Reward. Governments and ministries of health need to reward doc-tors for collaborating with ethnomedical practitioners. Within the job description for rural doctors should be an objective of collabo-rating with ethnomedical practitioners, and if they do this, then salary increments could be given. The same agencies also need to reward ethnomedical practitioners for their services to health. Some incentives are training courses, equipment, and transportation (such as bikes). Ceremonies, certificates, and diplomas are inexpen-sive but prestigious and valued rewards.

For example, under the leadership of Paul Hartenberger, USAID in Bolivia financed the travel of two Kallawaya herbalists to the Inter-national Congress of Traditional Medicine in Mexico as a reward. One of them, Mario Salcedo (who was president of Bolivia's ethno-medicine society), describes this experience as the high point of his career. Moreover, USAID's gesture firmly set the policy that herbal-ists are important in health development projects and that they will be rewarded with resources. As another example, Project Concern in Bolivia rewarded productive community health workers with herbal books, lanterns, and blackboards.

A substantial reward for ethnomedical practitioners is to receive free training in modern medicine and public health matters. Joint training between doctors and healers is also a way to begin collaboration between both medicines. What works best is to provide a short training course with simple objectives that need to be carried out in the community, and if participants accomplish these, then they can participate in another level of training.

Health Records: Key to Articulation

One major step to achieve effective collaboration between biomedical and ethnomedical practitioners is through health records. Files on patients are needed to determine what therapies have been used by biomedical and ethnomedical practitioners so that the results can be determined and a continuity maintained throughout the total therapeutic process. In rural Bolivia, doctors and nurses keep records of treatments, but these records are neither available to patients nor transferred. When patients switch treatments or are referred to another practitioner, there is limited opportunity for coordinating treatments because peasants are infrequently told the diagnosis and they seldom remember what the prescriptions were.

One solution is to issue health cards. When notaries or nurses register a child on its first visit to the clinic, they should issue a health card with entries for vaccination shots, nutritional status, diseases, and treatments. Under the category of treatments should be a blank for the name of the midwife who delivered the child and entries for names of ethnomedical practitioners, along with prescribed treatments. Because many ethnomedical practitioners can neither read nor write, the community health workers should fill in this information. For any medical treatment, cards would be required, thereby reinforcing their necessity. Although Bolivians rarely lose records when they have them, delay in treatment sometimes results when patients get sick away from their villages and must return to get their cards before they are treated. Exceptions are made, but people need be trained to carry health cards with them, along with their carnets of identity.

Advantages of such cards are that the various biomedical and ethnomedical practitioners can review a patient's medical history regarding efficacy of the different therapies. Although ethnomedical practitioners frequently cannot read, symbols can be used to indicate certain problems: a red star for malnutrition, a white star for tuberculosis, and a black circle for birth complications. Community health workers serve as coordinators of health cards in that they distribute them to individuals or families and assist them in recording the information. Of importance, community health workers must train and assist ethnomedical practitioners to make entries for their patients. When ethnomedical practitioners refuse, forget, or are unable to do this, community health workers can fill in the information by proxy. They can get this information from patients, their relatives, and other ethnomedical practitioners.

Ethnomedical practitioners participate in record keeping with health cards when they realize the benefits for their patients and themselves. Benefits for patients are that ineffective therapies need not be repeated and that treatments are complementary. Benefits for ethnomedical practitioners are that health cards make them aware of patients' illnesses and prior treatments, provide information about patients' lives and families, and record therapies for them to evaluate their effectiveness. Community health workers periodically review patients' health cards to evaluate patients' health and therapeutic effectiveness, and they communicate this information to ethnomedical practitioners to improve their practices.

Because ethnomedical practitioners object to record keeping for fear of being controlled by the biomedical bureaucracy, it is essential that health cards only be used for ways to improve and coordinate therapies of patients. These records should not serve as documents to resolve conflicts in accusations of malpractice. Ethnomedical practitioners can then be told that when they provide the necessary information it will not be used against them in any way except to evaluate the effectiveness of their therapies and that this information is for them, their patients, and for referrals.

Failure to standardize cards creates problems. In the Department of Oruro, Project Concern distributed health cards, called *carpetas,* through nurses and community health workers, who gave them to families and helped them fill in the information. After spending two years and $12,000, Project Concern's efforts were thwarted when UNICEF distributed a different type of health card in the same area and confused peasants as to which cards were valid (Wally Chastain, pers. com. 1991). To avoid this, coordination of health agencies and ministries is necessary to standardize health cards throughout the country. Standardized cards facilitate the coordination of health workers and diminish confusion, especially when peasants travel and visit health practitioners in other regions.

The project Save the Children implemented an efficient file system at the family level for peasants of Province Inquisivi, Bolivia (Bruce Harris, pers. com. 1988). Sixty-four community health workers register vital events (birth, marriage, death, nutrition, sicknesses, and injuries) and treatments for 20,000 people. This information is sent to a *supervisor del campo* (supervisor of the village), an auxiliary nurse who supports community health workers in six villages. The supervisors relay the medical information to a *coordinador* (coordinator), a public health nurse or medical doctor who supports five supervisors. The coordinators enter the information into a computer with a Database III program. This program assists health workers to keep track of people's health. When community health workers learn that someone is pregnant, they inform the supervisor, who passes it along to the coordinator, who enters it into the computer, which schedules three prenatal checkups. Community health workers do the same for deaths, except that causes are entered, and for marriages so that a new file can be entered. The computer program organizes people according to nutritional standards, diseases, and treatments.

Referral: Articulation in Action

When health cards are used, referral is greatly facilitated because biomedical and ethnomedical practitioners can study the results of each others' practices and patients' clinical history. (Unfortunately, doctors in the Department of Oruro often did not refer to health cards [Wally Chastain, pers. com. 1991].) Patients frequently visit both types of practitioners, often first one and then, if not satisfied, the other. Dissatisfaction is the motive most frequently given for changing therapists. A significant number of patients consult with biomedical and ethnomedical practitioners simultaneously. Since doctors rarely refer patients to healers and because referral is one way up the biomedical ladder, they need training on when and how to refer patients to ethnomedical practitioners. Doctors must learn to recognize psychosocial and cultural illnesses, which ethnomedical practitioners effectively treat. Doctors need to be trained to work with midwives to assist them in referrals of difficult deliveries rather than competing with them when the skills of midwives are adequate.

Ethnomedical healers infrequently refer patients to doctors and nurses because they often lose patients. Doctors discourage patients from returning to ethnomedical practitioners by discrediting their therapy. When midwives refer mothers with complications to doctors, they rarely get credit for their roles in births of the babies (Gretchen Berggren, pers. com. 1990). One solution to this problem is exemplified by Dr. Galbel in northeast Brazil, who brought midwives into the hospital and supervised their deliveries (Richard Guidotti, pers. com. 1990). Participation ensures the autonomy of the client-patient relationship by allowing the ethnomedical healer to be represented throughout the therapy. Where ethnomedical healers are forbidden to practice in hospitals, they naturally perceive the doctors and nurses of these institutions as enemies and competitors, perceptions certainly not conducive to referral and integration.

A major concern of ethnomedical practitioners is that doctors and nurses rarely, if ever, refer patients to them, which leads ethnomedical healers to conclude that doctors are superior, that they do not recognize the role of ethnomedicine, and that referrals are only one-way. Doctors need to be able to distinguish between worthless ethnomedical practices and those that cure in response to physical or psychosocial causes. Since health records provide indices of what has and has not worked for patients, community health workers can assist doctors and nurses in evaluating ethnomedical information on health cards.

Ethnomedical practitioners must be included in health programs and brought into the communication system of referrals by health cards and training courses. They need training in how to make diagnoses and where to make referrals. In the Department of Oruro, Bolivia, ethnomedical and biomedical practitioners are trained in a series of one-week courses and three weeks of practical supervision concerning medical protocols of how you deal with patients, recognition of symptoms, treatments, and referrals. Doctors, nurses, community health workers, (some of whom are ethnomedical practitioners), midwives, herbalists and shamans attend these meetings. Participants learn whether patients' needs are psychosocial therapy by shamans, medicinal plants from herbalists, delivery by midwives, primary care by community health workers or auxiliary nurses, surgery by doctors at the regional hospital, or referral to specialists in Oruro. Patients are brought into these training sessions for joint diagnoses and prescribed treatments by biomedical and ethnomedical practitioners.

Another way to assist ethnomedical practitioners in identifying complicated cases is by charts outlining potential problems and what to do. Because certain illnesses are culturally perceived, these charts need to be made out for each region.

Ethnomedical Healers and Collaboration

There are ways by which to encourage ethnomedical healers to collaborate with doctors and nurses: specifically, records, associations, recognition, and retraining.

Records. As discussed above, ethnomedical practitioners need to keep track of their patients and treatments by recording the patient's name, diagnosis, and treatment in notebooks on a daily basis. Mario Salcedo does this, and he also writes the formulas of his herbal prescriptions. Salcedo is instrumental in recovering much herbal folklore, rapidly disappearing as old-time herbalists die. Many ethnomedical practitioners who are promoters keep logs to catalog information on ethnomedicine, especially on medicinal plants. At health posts, nurses dry and press the plants to show to other practitioners. When biomedical and ethnomedical practitioners collaborate and share medicinal information, a collegial spirit develops that motivates them to further cooperation.

A prevalent problem in record keeping in Bolivia is that many ethnomedical practitioners are sensitive to being illiterate. Community health workers or a member of the *Comité de Salud* can assist by periodically questioning them as to their patients and treatments, and later recording this information. As an analogy, members of education committees in rural communities of Bolivia assist teachers in primary schools by translating from Spanish to the Aymara language in classrooms. Likewise, members of health committees in the villages can assist ethnomedical practitioners in recording treatments.

Anthropologists can assist ethnomedical practitioners in recording their therapies since they employ participant observation as a method to understand the social and cultural context of ethnomedicine (see Bastien 1987; Crandon-Malamud 1991). With this detailed observation and subsequent analysis, anthropologists can explain the psychosocial, ecological, and cultural functions of these therapies to biomedical practitioners. Collaborating with doctors, anthropologists can decipher harmful ethnomedical practices and suggest culturally sensitive ways of transforming maladaptive practices to salubrious health measures. This transformation involves an in-depth understanding of ethnomedicine, biomedicine, and culture change, which necessitates collegial collaboration among social scientists and biomedical and ethnomedical practitioners.

A more technologically sophisticated approach to record keeping is that proposed by ethnobiologist Dr. Conrad Gorinsky (1990): ethnomedical practitioners are trained to use "native-friendly" computers to enter information. About the size of a book and covered with plastic, these computers have graphics and digitilized screens with symbols that can be used as keyboards to designate entries. Gorinsky has trained herbalists in the Amazon to use similar computers for information about medicinal plants. Through Telelink and Chatbox, Gorinsky communicates from London with these herbalists. Chatbox is a group of handicapped children in London trained in computer communication especially for the use of "bulletin board" programs.

For most ethnomedical practitioners, information is mentally retained and orally transmitted. Written texts are inadequate means of storing and retrieving this information (Gorinsky 1990). In Bolivia, medical records are stored in warehouses and infrequently used for data analysis because of the time needed to sort out the information. Computer records and programs can sort and analyze information efficiently and rapidly. Data processing, local data bases, and links to other data bases are now the plow of communication systems. This technology can be used to link biomedical and ethnomedical practitioners throughout the world.

As a possible example, an African suffers from an insect bite for which local herbalists have no cure. The community health worker enters a description of the insect and information about the symptoms of the bite into a computer. This information is sent to computerized data bases in the Amazon to see if they have some native antidote; in London to see if biologists, entomologists, and pharmacologists at the University of London can prescribe some synthetic drug; and in New York, where a retired doctor, plugged into the network for humanitarian reasons, recalls that he was bitten by a similar bug while in Vietnam, where natives cured it with frog skins. Through the computer, all of the data obtained from these information resources is returned to Africa, where it is used to cure the person and add to the local data base of health care.

The cost of a computerized record system is high, and unless subsidized by international agencies, is unaffordable for developing countries. In addition to health care, efficiency, and collaboration, one scientific advantage is that a computerized system facilitates recording fast-disappearing ethnoscientific data. Within tropical forests of Brazil, species of plants and animals and tribes of people are becoming extinct yearly. The ethnomedicine of these tribes is also being lost, much of which is knowledge of herbal medicines that has been accumulated over centuries. With computerized data bases, pharmaceutical companies have access to this information for research on new drugs and accordingly should share some cost in implementing computer systems.

It should be mandatory that pharmaceutical companies grant patents and provide remuneration to ethnomedical practitioners and communities for products derived from these peoples' ethnomedicines. Rarely, if ever, have ethnic groups been given any part of the profits derived from medicinal plants used for research or marketed by pharmaceutical companies. As a good example, Kallawaya herbalists have furnished Bolivian pharmaceutical companies around fifty medicinal plants, from which pharmaceutical products have been manufactured. Yet, this ethnic group has not received any remuneration. As equitable way of compensation, a percentage of the profit could be granted to the ethnic group and the money used for needed communal projects, such as an herbal college, road, school, or tractor, which ones to be decided by community members.

Associations. One solution to the danger that ethnomedical healers will be subsumed by and considered inferior in the dominant medical system is for them to form associations. Previously, ethnomedical practitioners maintained closely knit associations with each other through kinship ties, and they guarded, but shared, esoteric knowledge. The function of these groups was to pass along the information to qualified people. Criteria for qualification included kinship and personal ties, practicing as apprentices, and group approval. Members of the group recognized degrees of skill among practitioners. Sick people asked members of their family, who asked other patients who the successful healers were. As illustrated in chapter 3, until 1950, Kallawaya herbalists maintained group identity and became world famous by careful training of apprentices and monitoring for total quality control. By implicit agreement and by inheritance of knowledge and practices, these herbalists distributed plants across South America.

More recently, urbanization has changed ethnic and community monitoring: Kallawayas have settled in cities, formed other associations, and lost close contact with communities in the Kallawaya region as well as some of their herbal tradition. Older herbalists complain that young practioners learn healing skills too rapidly from books without practice. Old-time herbalists complain that their tradition and reputation is being eroded by the frauds of the untrained. Patients do not know who the skilled herbalists are, because so many people call themselves Kallawaya herbalists. Doctors become alarmed at cases of herbal malpractice and then generalize that all Kallawayas are unskilled.

In response, Kallawaya herbalists have formed an association of ethnomedical practitioners, independent of the government and the dominant medical establishment, which evaluates members and their practices and represents them in public and in negotiation with doctors and politicians. Similar associations were discussed in chapter 5 for community health workers in Oruro and in chapter 4 for healers in Zaire (Last 1986). These associations are flexible to allow for the dynamic aspects of alternative medical systems, which function according to principles of folklore. As guilds once did, ethnomedical associations monitor aspiring herbalists to put some check on those ill-prepared. While this is no guarantee against malpractice, it is, along with patients' recommendations, still the best criteria for selecting healers, whether in bio- or ethnomedicine.

These associations, rather than ministries of health, certify and publicize who the qualified practitioners are. The majority of ethnomedical practitioners do not want to be licensed by doctors who they fear will use biomedical standards to evaluate ethnomedicine. They realize that licensing is a power procedure, giving control to those who do it. If ethnomedical practitioners need to be certified or licensed, then this should be done autonomously by themselves or the governing body of the ethnomedical association.

Recognition. Associations are also necessary to provide ethnomedical practitioners with recognition. Associations of midwives foster legitimacy for birth attendants. They periodically hold regional, national, and international congresses for exchanging information. As president of the ethnomedical medicine society in Bolivia, Mario Salcedo frequently writes articles on ethnomedicinal healing for La Paz newspapers. Representatives of this association also attended workshops on ways that both medicines can collaborate.

Ethnomedical practitioners also need to recognize the role of biomedicine in curing by accepting the limits of their efforts and knowing when to refer patients to other practitioners. This recognition is attained by allowing ethnomedical practitioners to observe the practice of doctors and nurses and by integrating clinics and hospitals. Examples provided in the chapters are from Navajo hospitals, where physicians and hand-tremblers jointly provide therapy for patients; from northeast Brazil, where midwives deliver babies, assisted by doctors; and from La Paz, where a woman physician, male homeopathologist, and Kallawaya herbalist practice together, administering herbs, drugs, and massages and performing minor operations.

Ethnographic and biomedical research is necessary to determine what ethnomedical practices are potentially harmful. More research is needed on plants to determine therapeutic efficacy and levels of toxicity so that herbalists become aware of the effects and dangers of plants. Wanting recognition, ethnomedical practitioners can provide information about their therapies to be investigated by doctors and social scientists. Kallawaya herbalists historically guarded ethnobotanical information until around 1980, when they allowed ethnobotanists to study their plants so that this information would not be lost and also so that the curative and toxic effects of plants could be investigated. Ethnomedical healers are recognized more when they make their healing techniques known to doctors and nurses.

A problem persistent to ethnomedicine, as well as biomedicine, is that it is difficult to evaluate its effect. That there are harmful practices as well as other practices which have proven over time to be useful is evident, however. Since practices persist for many reasons— efficacy is only one—the task is to separate them out, at least to the extent of eliminating the harmful ones. For doctors and nurses, this task is enormously difficult because they tend to overemphasize physical efficacy and, until recently, underemphasize therapy for secondary purposes, such as abrogation of the sick role, social support, resolving conflict, spiritual renewal, and catharsis. In curing rituals of Kaata, Bolivia, diviners symbolically feed the earth shrines of the three production zones on the mountain with an implicit understanding that the mountain will feed and provide them with nutrients for a complete body (see Bastien 1978). This ritual perdures because it is environmentally and nutritionally adaptive. Although anthropologists realize this, biomedical practitioners have little patience with this ritual therapy for patients with serious illnesses. A solution suitable to all (ethnomedicine, biomedicine, and environment) is for (1) practitioners to discontinue harmful practices, (2) practitioners to realize therapies are useful in many ways, and (3) patients to receive joint treatment by biomedical and ethnomedical practitioners when needed.

Retraining. Ethnomedical practitioners need retraining in many aspects of biomedicine. Advances in medicine should be accessible to all medical systems, and it is the responsibility of biomedical personnel to make this information available to ethnomedical practitioners. Whether ethnomedical healers incorporate this knowledge into their practices is their responsibility, but they should be given the opportunity. Consider the example of neonatal tetanus, discussed in chapter 8, a terrible disease that kills upwards of 441,000 infants a year and can be eliminated by tetanus toxoid, a highly successful (90 percent) antigen. To prevent these deaths, midwives need to be retrained to administer antiseptically clean deliveries and to insist that mothers be vaccinated with the tetanus toxoid. Herbalists can be taught either to give injections or to educate patients about vaccinations. Almost all ethnomedical practitioners need instruction in aseptic practices.

Illustrated in chapter 5, a highly effective way to retrain ethnomedical practitioners has been through the role of community health workers. A large proportion of community health workers in Bolivia and in other parts of the world are ethnomedical practitioners who want to learn about biomedicine. The key to success in Bolivia is that they are selected by members of the community, especially the women, and not just the leaders, and are accountable to them. Supervised by doctors, community health workers remain independent of them and have formed an association. The Ministry of Health provides them with a series of two-week workshops, rudimentary medical supplies, and supervision. As community health workers, midwives, herbalists, and shamans have learned and adopted curative first-aid practices, diagnoses, and referral techniques. Community health workers who are not ethnomedical practitioners assume responsibility for coordinating efforts of biomedical and ethnomedical practitioners.

Essential to the success of the Oruro community health-worker program are workshops provided for biomedical personnel, ethnomedical practitioners, and CHWs, where they discuss differences and strategies for public health measures and rural health-delivery programs. Although these workshops generate some disagreement, they provide opportunities for friendship and dialogue.

In sum, doctors and nurses need to *recognize, respect,* and *reward* ethnomedical practitioners. Pharmaceutical companies need to provide monetary *recompense* for medicines derived from ethnomedical sources. Ethnomedical practitioners need to strive for *reunion,*

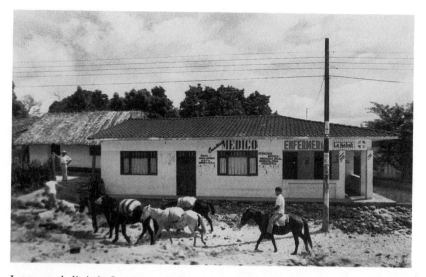

Integrated clinic in Samaypata, where doctors, nurses, herbalists, and shamans are effectively incorporating biomedicine and ethnomedicine in their practices.

recognition, retraining, and *referral.* These are the required "R"s for successful collaboration between biomedical and ethnomedical practitioners. The goals are holistic medicine and world health for all. At a time in history with a universal and massive conjuncture of cultures (people coming together in space and time), doctors and *curanderos,* psychiatrists and shamans, herbalists and pharmacists, obstetricians and midwives, vaccinators and hexers can interact in a cultural and biological struggle against the finitude and forces of nature.

Although collaboration is difficult, it has begun in Bolivia. One final example is that between a doctor and shaman in the Department of Oruro. Edgar Francken is a Belgian cleric-doctor, who because of his religious affiliations was at first adamantly opposed to the use of ethnomedical practitioners, especially shamans, in his practice. After attending several workshops on ethnomedicine in Oruro, Francken recognized the importance of collaboration and invited shamans and herbalists to work with him at the hospital of Totora, where he was director. He gained the respect of herbalists and shamans throughout the region. When his son was dying of cancer, a leading shaman asked Francken to operate. Even though his son died shortly after the operation, the shaman invited

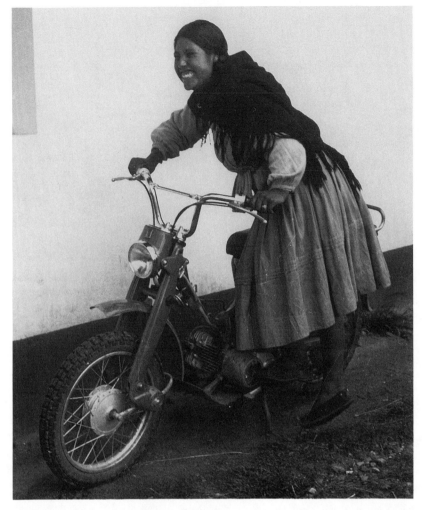

Motorbike is used by community health worker to visit distant communities in the Altiplano.

Francken to the funeral and afterward embraced him, thanking him publicly for his efforts, and told those present that he was a good healer. Later, the shaman asked to learn about anatomy and Francken presented him with an illustrated book on body parts (Velasco, pers. com. 1987).

Edgar Francken's efforts were rewarded in 1986 when he asked that the *jilacatas* (leaders) of the communities, in the zone of Totora (about 7,000 people, with seventeen CHWs), provide more than manual labor for their annual *mit'a* contribution to the district.

Mit'a is an ancient Andean tradition that literally means "one's turn at work" and refers to manual labor obligations such as rebuilding bridges and repairing roads. The *jilacatas* agreed to have all the children vaccinated by community health workers. At the first of the year, they presented Francken with a list of all the children vaccinated. This was a milestone in that *jilacatas* used *mit'a* as an institutional mechanism for public health projects. And it happened mainly because Edgar Francken had gained the respect of the native practitioners, who in turn had influenced the *jilacatas* (Grisel Saenz, pers. com. 1987).

Similar types of collaboration between biomedical and ethnomedical practitioners are possible and needed to provide integrated health programs throughout the world.

References

Abercrombie, Thomas
  1986 "The Politics of Sacrifice: An Andean Cosmology in Action." Ph.D. diss., University of Chicago.
Adams, Richard N.
  1952 "Un Análisis de las Creencias y Prácticas Médicas en un Pueblo Indígena de Guatemala." *Publicaciones Especiales del Instituto Indigenista Nacional.* Publicación 17. Guatemala.
  1981 "Natural Selection, Energetics, and 'Cultural Materialism'." *Current Anthropology* 22 (6): 603–24.
Ademuwagun, Zaccheus, J. A. Ayoade, D. M. Warren, and I. Harrison, eds.
  1979 *African Therapeutic Systems.* Los Angeles: Crossroads Press.
Aitken, I. W., T. K. Kargbo, and A. M. Gba-Kamara
  1985 "Planning a Community-Oriented Midwifery Service for Sierra Leone." *World Health Forum* 6 (2): 110–14.
Akerele, Olayiwola
  1983 "Which Way for Traditional Medicine?" *World Health: The Magazine of the World Health Organization* (June): 3–4.
  1984 "WHO's Traditional Medicine Programme: Progress and Perspectives." *World Health Organization Chronicle* 38 (2): 76–81.
  1987 "The Best of Both Worlds: Bringing Traditional Medicine up to Date." *Social Science and Medicine* 24 (2) :177–81.
Albo, Xavier
  1979 *Achacachi: Medio Siglo de Lucha Campesina. Cuadernos de Investigación.* La Paz: CIPCA.
  1985 *Desafíos de la Solidaridad Aymara.* La Paz: CIPCA.
  _____, A. Godínez, K. Libermann, and F. Pifarré
  1989 *Para Comprender las Culturales Rurales en Bolivia.* La Paz: MEC, CIPCA, UNICEF.
Alisjahbana, A., R. Peeters, and A. Meheus
  1986 "Traditional Birth Attendants Can Identify Mothers and Infants at Risk." *World Health Forum* 7 (3): 240–47.
Allport, Gordon
  1937 *Personality. A Psychological Interpretation.* New York: Henry Holt.
Alvarado, Anita L.
  1978 "Utilization of Ethnomedical Practitioners and Concepts within the Framework of Western Medicine." In *Modern Medicine and Medical Anthropology in the United States-Mexico Border Population,* edited by Boris Velimirovic, 17–21. Washington, D.C.: Pan American Health Organization.
Ampofo, Daniel A., David D. Nicholas, Mavis B. Amonoo-Acquah, Samuel Ofosu-Amaah, and Alfred K. Neumann
  1977 "The Training of Traditional Birth Attendants in Ghana: Experience of the Danfa Rural Health Project." *Tropical and Geographical Medicine* 29:197–203.

Anonymous
  1991 *Qualitative Research on Knowledge, Attitudes, and Practices Related to Wom-
         en's Reproductive Health, Cochabamba, Bolivia.* Working Paper no. 9.
         MotherCare Project, REACH. Arlington: John Snow.
Anderson, W. Timothy, and David T. Helm
  1979 "The Physician-Patient Encounter: A Process of Reality Negotiation."
         In *Patients, Physicians, and Illness*, edited by E. Jaco, 259–71. New York:
         Free Press.
Arellano López, Jorge
  1978 "La Cultura Mollo: Ensay de Síntesis Arqueológica." *Pumapunku*
         12:87–113.
Arnold, Denise
  1988 "Matrilineal Practices in a Patrilineal Setting: Rituals and Mataphors
         of Kinship in an Andean Ayllu." Ph.D. diss., University of London.
  1900 "The House of Earth-bricks and Inka-stones: Gender, Memory and
         Cosmos in Ayllu Qaqachaka." Paper presented at Cornell University.
  1990a " 'Scattering the seeds' ": Shared Thoughts on Some Songs to the
         Food Crops from an Andean Ayllu." With Domingo Jiménez Arukipa
         and Juan de Dios Yapita Moya. In *The Spoken Word: Language, Discourse,
         and Society in the Andes.* Edited by Rosaleen Howard-Malverde. Latin
         American Institute Monographs. London: University of London.
Ayala Benitez, Alfonso, and Gloria Torrico Espinoza
  1988 "Tétanus Neonatal: Estudio de Tres Años en el Hospital de Niños de
         Montero." unpub. ms.
Baer, Hans A.
  1987 "Divergence and Convergence in Two Systems of Manual Medicine:
         Osteopathy and Chiropractic in the United States." *Medical Anthropol-
         ogy Quarterly* 1:176–93.
Bahr, Donald M., Juan Gregorio, David Lopez, and Alberto Alvarez
  1974 *Piman Shamanism and Staying Sickness.* Tucson: University of Arizona
         Press.
Bancroft-Hunt, Norman
  1981 *The Indians of the Great Plains.* London: Orbis Publishing Limited.
Bandelier, Adolf
  1904 "Aboriginal Trephining in Bolivia." *American Anthropologist* 6:440–46.
Banerji, D.
  1978 "Place of the Indigenous and Wester Systems of Medicine in Health
         Services of India." Paper presented at the Ninth World Congress of
         Sociology, Uppsala, Sweden.
Barnouw, Victor
  1985 *Culture and Personality.* Homewood, Ill.: The Dorsey Press.
Bastien, Joseph W.
  1973 *Qollahuaya Rituals: An Ethnographic Account of the Symbolic Relations of
         Man and Land in an Andean Village.* Ithaca: Cornell University Latin
         American Studies Program.
  1978 *Mountain of the Condor: Metaphor and Ritual in an Andean Ayllu.* Ameri-
         can Ethnological Society Monograph 64. St. Paul: West Publishing
         Company. (Reissued by Waveland Press, 1985.)
  1980 "Rosinta, Rats, and the River: Bad Luck Is Banished in Andean
         Bolivia." In *Unspoken Worlds: Women's Religious Lives in Non-Western Cul-
         tures,* edited by Nancy Falk and Rita Gross, 260–74. New York: Harper
         and Row.

1982 "Herbal Curing by Qollahuaya Andeans," *Journal of Ethnopharmacology* 6:13–28.

1982a "Exchange between Andean and Western Medicine." *Social Science and Medicine* 16:795–803.

1983 "Pharmacopeia of Qollahuaya Andeans." *Journal of Ethnopharmacology* 8:97–111.

1983a *Las plantas Medicinales de los Kallawayas.* Oruro: Proyecto Concern.

1985 "Qollahuaya-Andean Body Concepts: A Topographical-Hydraulic Model of Physiology." *American Anthropologist* 87:595–611.

1987 *Healers of the Andes: Kallawaya Herbalists and Their Medicinal Plants.* Salt Lake City: University of Utah Press.

1987a "Cross-cultural Communication between Doctors and Peasants in Bolivia." *Social Science and Medicine* 24:1109–18.

1988 *Cultural Perceptions of Neonatal Tetanus and Programming Implications, Bolivia.* Resources for Child Health Project. Arlington: REACH, John Snow, Inc.

1988a "Shaman contra Enfermero en los Andes Bolivianos." *Allpanchis* 31:163–97.

1989 "A Shamanistic Curing Ritual of the Bolivian Aymara." *Journal of Latin American Lore* 15 (1): 73–94.

1990 "Community Health Workers in Bolivia: Adapting to Traditional Roles in the Andean Community." *Social Science and Medicine* 30:281–88.

———, W. Mahler, M. Reinecke, W. Robinson, J. Zalles, and Yongua Shu

1990 "Testing of Anti-HIV Compounds from Bolivian-Kallawaya Medicinal Plants." Paper presented at Second International Congress of Ethnobiology, October 22–28, Kunming, China.

Behrhorst, Carroll

1972 "Report on Survey Trip through Africa and Asia." Brunswick, Georgia: MAP International. Mimeo.

1974 "The Chimaltenango Development Project, Guatemala." In *Contact* #19, Christian Medical Commission. Geneva: World Council of Churches.

1975 "The Chimaltenango Development Project in Guatemala." In *Health by the People,* edited by Kenneth W. Newell, 30–52. Geneva: World Health Organization.

1983 "Introduction." In *Health in the Guatemalan Highlands,* edited by Ulli Steltzer, xi-xxxv. Seattle: University of Washington Press.

Belcher, Donald W., Alfred K. Neumann, Frederick K. Wurapa, David D. Nicholas, and Samuel Ofosu-Amaah

1975 "The Role of Health Survey Research in Maternal and Child/Family Planning Programmes: Danfa Project, Ghana." *Journal of Tropical Pediatrics and Environmental Child Health* 21(4):173–77.

———, Alfred K. Neumann, Samuel Ofosu-Amaah, David D. Nicholas, and S. N. Blumenfeld

1978 "Attitudes towards Family Size and Family Planning in Rural Ghana—Danfa Project: 1972 Survey Findings." *Journal of Biosocial Science* 10:59–79.

Bell, D. E., and M. R. Reich, eds.

1988 *Health, Nutrition, and Economic Crises: Approaches to Policy in the Third World.* Dover, Mass.: Auburn House Publishing Co.

Benson, Herbert, and M.D. Epstein
1975   "The Placebo Effect: A Neglected Asset in the Care of Patients." *Journal of the American Medical Association* 232:1225–27.
Berger, Peter L., and Thomas Luckmann
1967   *The Social Construction of Reality.* Garden City: Anchor Books.
Bergin, Allen E.
1971   "The Evaluation of Therapeutic Outcomes." In *Handbook of Psychotherapy and Behavior Change*, edited by Allen Bergin and Sol L. Garfield, 217–70. New York: John Wiley and Sons.
Berman, P. A., D. R. Gwatkin, and S. E. Burger
1987   "Community-Based Health Workers: Head Start or False Start towards Health for All?" *Social Science and Medicine* 25 (5): 443–59.
Bibeau, Gilles
1982   "New Legal Rules for an Old Art of Healing: The Case of Zairian Healers' Associations." *Social Science and Medicine* 16:1843–49.
Billington, W. R., H. F. Welbourn, K. C. N. Wandera, and A. W. Sengendo
1963   "Custom and Child Health in Buganda. III. Pregnancy and Childbirth." *Tropical and Geographical Medicine* 15:134–37.
Blanchet, Teresa
1989   *Perceptions of Childhood Diseases and Attitudes towards Immunization among Slum Dwellers in Dhaka, Bangladesh.* Arlington, Va.: REACH, John Snow, Inc.
Bourne, P.
1987   "Beyond the Barefoot Doctor: The Unfilled Promise of Primary Health Care." *Development International* 1 (3): 32–35.
Bravo, Carlos
1918   "El Callahuaya." *Boletín de la Sociedad Geográfica de La Paz* 47:167–72.
Brock, D. Heyward, ed.
1984   *The Culture of Biomedicine: Studies in Science and Culture*, vol. 1. Newark: University of Delaware Press.
Brown, Jack
1963   "Some Changes in Mexican Village Curing Practices Induced by Western Medicine." *América Indígena* 23:93–120.
Bryant, J. H.
1980   "WHO's Program of Health for All by the Year 2000: A Macrosystem for Health Policy Making—A Challenge to Social Science Research." *Social Science and Medicine* 14A (5):381–86.
Buechler, H., and J-M. Buechler
1971   *The Bolivian Aymara.* New York: Holt, Rinehart & Winston.
Buxton, Jean
1973   *Religion and Healing in Mandari.* Oxford: University of Oxford Press.
Buzzard, Shirley
1987   *Development Assistance and Health Programs: Issues of Sustainability.* AID Program Evaluation Discussion Paper no. 23. Washington, D.C.: USAID.
Carter, William
1965   *Aymara Communities and the Bolivian Agrarian Reform.* Monograph 24. Gainesville: University of Florida Press.
_____, and M. Mamani
1989   *Irpa Chico: Individuo y Communidad en la Cultura Aymara.* La Paz: Editorial "Juventud."

Catsambas, Thanos, and Susan Foster
1986 "Spending Money Sensibly: The Case of Essential Drugs." *Finance and Development* 23:29–32.
Chabot, H.T. J.
1984 "Primary Health Care Will Fail If We Do Not Change Our Approach." *The Lancet* 1:340–41.
Clifford, James
1988 *The Predicament of Culture.* Boston: Harvard University Press.
Cole, J.
1987 *Latin American Inflation: Theoretical Interpretations and Empirical Results.* New York: Praeger Publishers.
Coolidge, Mary R.
1975 *The Rain-Makers.* Santa Fe: William Gannon.
Coreil, Jeannine, and J. Dennis Mull.
1990 *Anthropology and Primary Health Care.* Boulder, Colo.: Westview Press.
Cosminsky, Sheila
1974 "The Role of Midwife in Middle America." Paper presented at the Forty-first International Congress of Americanists, September 2–7, Mexico City, Mexico.
1976 "Cross-Cultural Perspectives on Midwifery." In *Medical Anthropology,* edited by F. Grollig and H. Haley, 229–41. The Hague: Mouton.
1977 "Childbirth and Midwifery on a Guatemalan Finca." *Medical Anthropology Quarterly* 1 (Summer): 69–104.
1978 "Midwifery and Medical Anthropology." In *Modern Medicine and Medical Anthropology in the United States-Mexico Border Population,* edited by Boris Velimirovic, 116–26. Washington, D.C.: Pan American Health Organization.
————, and Ira Harrison
1984 *Traditional Medicine, vol. 2, 1976–1981: Current Research with Implications for Ethnomedicine, Ethnopharmacology, Maternal and Child Health, Mental Health and Public Health, an Annotated Bibliography of America, Latin America, and the Caribbean.* New York: Garland Publishing.
Crandon-Malamud, Libbet
1977 "Anthropological Report on the Montero Rural Health Project at the Community Level." Consultant's Report to USAID, Bolivian Mission, La Paz. Mimeo.
1980 "Changing Faces of the Achachillas: Medical Systems and Cultural Identity in a Highland Bolivian Village." Ph.D. diss., University of Massachusetts.
1983 "Grass Roots, Herbs, Promotors and Preventions: A Reevaluation of Contemporary International Health Care Planning, the Bolivian Case." *Social Science and Medicine* 17:1281–89.
1983a "Why Susto?" *Ethnology* 22:153–67.
1983b "Between Shamans, Doctors and Demons: Illness, Curing, and Cultural Identity Midst Culture Change." In *Third World Medicine and Social Change,* edited by John Morgan, 69–84. Lanham, Md.: University Press of America.
1987 "Medical Dialogue and the Political Economy of Medical Pluralism: A Case from Rural Highland Bolivia." *American Ethnologist* 13 (3): 463–88.
1991 *The Fat of Our Souls.* Berkeley: University of California Press.
Crankshaw, L. Crandon (see Crandon-Malamud)

de Kadt, E.
  1982 "Ideology, Social Policy, Health and Health Services: A Field of Complex Interactions." *Social Science and Medicine* 13C:203–11.
del Castillo, Jorge
  1983 "Situación de El Alto Norte." In *La Ciudad Prometida,* edited by Godofredo Sandoval Z. and M. Fernanda Sostres, 69. La Paz: ILDIS-SYSTEMA.
Dobbing, John
  1988 *Infant Feeding: Anatomy of a Controversy* 1973–1984. New York: Springer-Verlag.
Dobrin, Lyn
  1977 "Infant Formula Abuse: The Scandal." In *Breast versus Bottle: The Scandal of Infant Formula Promotion,* p. 1. Food Monitor Reprint. Garden City, N.Y.: World Hunger Year.
Donahue, J.
  1981 "Health Delivery in Rural Bolivia." In *Health in the Andes,* edited by J. Bastien and J. Donahue, 173–95. Washington, D.C.: American Anthropological Association.
  1990 "The Role of Anthropologists in Primary Health Care: Reconciling Professional and Community Interests." In *Anthropology and Primary Health Care,* edited by J. Coreil and J. D. Mull, 79–97. Boulder, Colo.: Westview Press.
Doore, Gary
  1988 *Shaman's Path: Healing, Personal Growth and Empowerment.* Boston: Shambhala Publishing.
Dreyfus, Hubert, and Paul Rabinow
  1983 *Michel Foucault: Beyond Structuralism and Hermeneutics.* Berkeley: University of California Press.
Duke, James
  1975 "Chemistry and Folk Medicine." In *Recent Advances in Phytochemistry,* vol. 9, edited by V. Runeckles, 83–100. New York: Plenum.
Dwivedi, K. N., and P. H. Rai
  1971 "The Training of Traditional Birth Attendants: A Broader Approach Is Needed." *International Journal of Health Education* 14:29–33.
Earls, J.
  1973 "La Organización del Poder en la Mitología Quechua." In *Ideología Mesiánica del Mundo Andino,* edited by Juan Ossio, 395–414. Lima: Morson.
Economist, The
  1985 "Primary Health Care Is Not Curing African Ills." May 31, 97–100.
Egbert, Lawrence, G. E. Battit, C. E. Welch, and M. Bartlett
  1964 "Reduction of Post-Operative Pain by Encouragement and Instruction of Patient." *New England Journal of Medicine* 270(16): 825–27.
Eisenberg, Leon
  1977 "Disease and Illness: Distinctions between Professional and Popular Ideas of Sickness." *Culture, Medicine and Psychiatry* 1:9–23.
Ekunwe, E.
  1984 " 'Standing orders'—A Powerful Tool in Primary Care." *World Health Forum* 5 (1): 19–23.
Eliade, Mircea
  1987 "Shamanism: An Overview." In *Encyclopedia of Religion,* vol. 13, edited by M. Eliade, 202–7. New York: Macmillan Publishing Company.

Engel, George
   1977 "The Need for a New Medical Model: A Challenge for Biomedicine."
       Science 196:129–36.
Evaluación Integral del Sector de Salud en Bolivia.
   1978 La Paz: USAID.
Fabrega, Horacio, Jr.
   1977 "Group Differences in the Structure of Illness." *Culture, Medicine and
       Psychiatry* 1:379–94
   _____, and Daniel Silver
   1973 *Illness and Shamanistic Curing in Zinacantan.* Stanford: Stanford Univer-
       sity Press.
Fathalla, Mahmood, K. Bhasker Rao, Kelsey A. Harrison, and Barbara Kwast
   1986 "Prevention of Maternal Mortality." *World Health Forum* 7:50–55.
Favin, M., R. Steinglass, and C. Betts
   1991 *Eliminating Neonatal Tetanus as a Public Health Problem in Santa Cruz
       Department, Bolivia.* REACH. Arlington, Virginia: John Snow.
Finkler, Kaja
   1981 "Dissident Religious Movements in the Service of Women's Power."
       Sex Roles: A Journal of Research 7:481–95.
   1985 *Spiritualist Healers in Mexico: Successes and Failures, Alternative Therapeu-
       tics.* New York: Bergin and Garvey Publishers.
Finnerman, Ruthbeth D.
   1989 "Tracing Home-Based Health Care Change in an Andean Indian
       Community." *Medical Anthropology Quarterly* 2:162–79.
Foster, George M.
   1958 "Problems in Intercultural Health Programs." Memorandum to the
       Committee on Preventative Medicine and Social Science Research.
       Washington, D.C.: Social Science Research Council.
   1977 "Medical Anthropology and International Health Planning." *Social
       Science and Medicine* 11:527–34.
   1978 "Hippocrates' Latin American Legacy: 'Hot' and 'Cold' in Contempo-
       rary Folk Medicine." In *Colloquia in Anthropology,* edited by R. K.
       Wetherington, 3–19. Dallas: Southern Methodist University.
   1987 "On the Origin of Humoral Medicine in Latin America." *Medical
       Anthropology Quarterly* 1:355–93.
   _____, and Barbara G. Anderson
   1978 *Medical Anthropology.* New York: John Wiley and Sons.
Foucault, Michel
   1975 *The Birth of the Clinic: An Archaeology of Medical Perception,* translated by
       A. M. Sheridan Smith. New York: Vintage/Random House.
Frank, Jerome D.
   1974 *Persuasion and Healing.* New York: Schocken Books.
Frankenberg, R.
   1978 "Allopathic Medicine, Profession and Capitalist Ideology in India."
       Paper presented at the Ninth World Congress of Sociology, Uppsala,
       Sweden.
Freud, Sigmund
   1933 "The Dissection of the Psychical Personality." In *Collected Works.*
       Standard edition. Vol. 22:57–80. London: Hogarth Press, reprint 1964.
Fromm, Erich
   1955 *The Sane Society.* New York: Rinehart.

Gaines, A. D., and R. A. Hahn
1985 *Physicians of Western Society.* Boston: D. Reidel.

Galazka, Arthur, and George Stroh
1986 *Neonatal Tetanus: Guidelines on the Community-Based Survey on Neonatal Tetanus Mortality.* Geneva: WHO.

Garrison, V.
1974 *Folk Healers and Community Mental Health Program Planning.* Informal Progress Report on NIMH Grant, MH 22563-01. Washington, D.C.: NIMH.
1977 "Doctor, *Espiritista,* or Psychiatrist?: Health- Seeking Behavior in a Puerto Rican Neighborhood of New York City." *Medical Anthropology* 1 (2):65-180.

Gill, Derek G.
1978 "Limitations upon Choice and Constraints over Decision- Making in Doctor-Patient Exchanges." In *The Doctor-Patient Relationship in the Changing Health Scene,* edited by Eugene B. Gallagher, 141-54. DHEW Publication No. (NIH) 78-183. Washington, D.C.: U.S. Department of Health, Education, and Welfare; Public Health Service, National Institute of Health.

Girault, Louis
1984 *Kallawaya: Guírisseurs Itinérants des Andes.* Paris: Mémoires ORSTOM.
1987 *Kallawayas: Curanderos Itinerantes de los Andes.* La Paz: UNICEF.
1988 *Rituales en las Regiones Andinas de Bolivia y Peru.* La Paz: Don Bosco.
1989 *Kallawaya: El Idioma Secreto de los Incas.* La Paz: UNICEF.

Gish, O.
1979 "The Political Economy of PHC and Health by the People: An Historical Explanation." *Social Science and Medicine* 16:1049-63.

Glasser, Morton
1977 "Psychiatric Cases in a Family Practice: Analysis of Outcomes." *Medical Anthropology* 1:55-73.

Glittenberg, Joann
1974 "Adapting Health Care to a Cultural Setting." *American Journal of Nursing* 74 (12): 2218-21.

Gonzales, N. S., and M. Behar
1966 "Childrearing Practices, Nutrition and Health Status." *Milbank Memorial Fund Quarterly* 44:77-96.

Good, B.
1977 "The Heart of What's the Matter: The Semantics of Illness in Iran." *Culture, Medicine and Psychiatry* 1:25-58.

Good, Charles
1987 *Ethnomedical Systems in Africa: Patterns of Traditional Medicine in Rural and Urban Kenya.* New York: The Guilford Press.

Gorinsky, Conrad
1990 "Sociocultural Studies of Folk Tradition in Relation to Ethnobiological Science." Paper presented at the Second International Congress of Ethnobiology, Kunming, China.

Green, Edward C.
1985 "Traditional Healers, Mothers and Childhood Diarrheal Disease in Swaziland: The Interface of Anthropology and Health Education." *Social Science and Medicine* 20 (3): 277-85.
1988 "Can Collaborative Programs between Biomedical and African

Indigenous Health Practitioners Succeed?" *Social Science and Medicine* 27 (11): 1125–30.

⸻, and Lydia Makhubu

1984 "Traditional Healers in Swaziland: Toward Improved Cooperation between the Traditional and Modern Health Sectors." *Social Science and Medicine* 18 (12): 1071–79

Greenburg, Linda

1982 "Midwife Training Programs in Highland Guatemala." *Social Science and Medicine* 16:1599–609.

Guaman Poma de Ayala, Felipe

1936 *Nueva Corónica y Buen Govierno.* Travaux et Mémoires de l'Institut d'Ethnologie, vol. 23. Paris.

Haire, Doris

1972 *The Cultural Warping of Childbirth.* A Special Report Prepared by the International Childbirth Education Association (Spring). Minneapolis: ICEA News.

Handelman, H.

1975 *Struggle in the Andes.* Austin: University of Texas Press.

Harner, Michael

1980 *The Way of the Shaman: A Guide to Power and Healing.* New York: Bantam Books.

Harrison, Ira, and Sheila Cosminsky

1976 *Traditional Medicine: Implications for Ethnomedicine, Ethnopharmacology, Maternal and Child Health, Mental Health and Public Health, an Annotated Bibliography of Africa, Latin America, and the Caribbean.* New York: Garland Publishing.

Harrison, J. L.

1974–75 "Traditional Healers: A Neglected Source of Health Manpower." In *Traditional Healers: Use and Non-Use in Health Care Delivery*, edited by I.E. Harrison and D. W. Dunlop, 5–16. East Lansing: The African Study Center.

Hatcher, Robert, F. Stewart, J. Trussell, D. Kuwal, and F. Guest

1992 *Contraceptive Technology.* 15th ed. New York: Irvington Publishers.

Haynes, Alfred M.

1978 "Medical Care and the Doctor-Patient Relationship." In *The Doctor-Patient Relationship in the Changing Health Scene*, edited by Eugene B. Gallagher, 39–96. DHEW Publication No. (NIH) 78–183. Washington, D.C.: U.S. Department of Health, Education, and Welfare; Public Health Service, National Institute of Health.

Heggenhougen, H. K.

1976 "Health Care for the 'Edge of the World': Indian Campesinos as Health Workers in Chimaltenango, Guatemala—A Discussion of the Behrhorst Program." Report prepared for the New School for Social Research, New York.

1984 "Will Primary Health Care Efforts Be Allowed to Succeed?" *Social Science and Medicine* 19 (3): 217–24.

Henry, J. L.

1982 "Possible Involvement of Endorphins in Altered States of Consciousness." *Ethos* 10 (4): 394–408.

Hobcraft, J., J. W. McDonald, and S. O. Rutstein

1983 "Child-Spacing Effects on Infant and Early Child Mortality." *Population Index* 49:585–618.

Holt, Keven H.
1990 "A Neuroanthropological Model of Ritual and the Modulation of Social Behavior." Honors Thesis in Anthropology, December 1990, University of Texas at Arlington.

Howard, Forrest H.
1951 "The Physiologic Position for Delivery." *Northwest Medicine* 50 (2): 98–100.
1958 "Delivery in the Physiologic Position." *Obstetrics and Gynecology* 11 (3): 318–22.

Hudson, Charles
1975 "Vomiting for Purity: Ritual Emesis in the Aboriginal Southeastern United States." In *Symbols and Society*, edited by Carole E. Hill, 93–102. Athens, Ga.: Southern Anthropological Society.

Hughes, Charles C.
1976 "Of Wine and Bottles, Old and New: An Anthropological Perspective on the 'New' Family Physician." In *Transcultural Health Care Issues and Conditions—Health Care Dimensions*, edited by Madelaine Leininger, 37–49. Philadelphia: F. A. Davis.

Illich, Ivan
1976 *Medical Nemesis: Expropriation of Health*. New York: Pantheon Books.

Imperato, Pascal James
1977 *African Medicine, Practices and Beliefs of the Bambara and Other Peoples*. Baltimore: New York Press.

Inui, Thomas, E. L. Yourtee, and J. W. Williamson
1976 "Improved Outcomes in Hypertensions after Physician Tutorials." *Annals of Internal Medicine* 84 (6): 646–51.

Isbell, Billie Jean
1978 *To Defend Ourselves: A View through an Andean Kaleidoscope*. Austin: University of Texas Press

Isenalumbe, A.E.
1990 "Integration of Traditional Birth Attendants into Primary Health Care." *World Health Forum* 11:192–98.

Iyun, F.
1989 "An Assessment of Rural Health Programme on Child and Maternal Care: The Ogbomoso Community Health Care Programme (CHCP), Oyo State, Nigeria." *Social Science and Medicine* 29 (8): 933–38.

Janowitz, Barbara, Sylvia Wallace, Galba Araujo, and Lorena Araujo
1985 "Referral by Traditional Birth Attendants in Northeast Brazil." *American Journal of Public Health* 75 (7): 745–48.

Janzen, John M.
1978 *The Quest for Therapy in Lower Zaire*. Berkeley: University of California Press.

Jeffery, Roger
1982 "Policies towards Indigenous Healers in Independent India." *Social Science and Medicine* 16 (21): 1835–41.

Jenkins, Carol, and Peter Heywood
1984 "A Method for Eliciting Beliefs about Food and Child Feeding in Papua New Guinea: The Machik Interview." *Papua New Guinea Medical Journal* 27:11–15.

Jerome, N. W., R. F. Kandel, and G. H. Pelto
1980 *Nutritional Anthropology: Contemporary Approaches to Diet and Culture*. Pleasantville, N. Y.: Redgrave.

Jilek, Wolfgang G.
1974 *Salish Indian Mental Health and Culture Change*. Toronto: Holt, Rinehart and Winston of Canada.
1982 "Altered States of Consciousness in North American Indian Ceremonials." *Ethos* 10 (4): 317–25.
Joralemon, Donald
1984 "The Role of Hallucinogenic Drugs and Sensory Stimuli in Peruvian Ritual Healing." *Culture, Medicine and Psychiatry* 8:399–430.
1986 "Performing Patient in Ritual Healing." *Social Science and Medicine* 23 (9): 841–45.
1990 "The Selling of the Shaman and the Problem of Informant Legitimacy." *Journal of Anthropological Research* 46 (2): 105–18.

———,
n.d. In Harm's Way: Shamans and Patients on the North Coast of Peru." Ms., Smith College, Northhampton, Mass.
Jordan, Brigitte
1975 "Two Studies in Medical Anthropology: Crosscultural Investigation of Birthing Systems in a Sociobiological Perspective." Ph.D. diss., University of California at Irvine.
1978 *Birth in Four Cultures: A Crosscultural Investigation of Childbirth in Yucatan, Holland, Sweden and the United States*. Canada: Eden Press.
1990 "Technology and the Social Distribution of Knowledge: Issues for Primary Health Care in Developing Countries." In *Anthropology and Primary Health Care*, edited by J. Coreil and J. D. Mull, 98–120. Boulder, Colo.: Westview Press.
Kane, S. M.
1982 "Holiness Ritual Fire Handling: Ethnographic and Psychophysiological Considerations." *Ethos* 10 (4): 369–84.
Karim, Wazir-Jahan
1984 "Malay Midwives and Witches." *Social Science and Medicine* 18 (2): 159–66.
Katon, Wayne, Arthur Kleinman, and Gary Rosen
1982 "Depression and Somatization: A Review, part 1." *The American Journal of Medicine* 72 (1): 127–35.
1982a "Depression and Somatization: A Review, part 2." *The American Journal of Medicine* 72 (2): 241–47.
Katz, R.
1982 "Accepting 'Boiling Energy': The Experience of !Kia-Healing among the !Kung." *Ethos* 10:344–68.
Kay, Margarita Artschwager, ed.
1982 *Anthropology of Human Birth*. Philadelphia: F. A. Davis.
Kelly, George A.
1955 *The Psychology of Personal Constructs*, vol. 1.: *A Theory of Personality*. New York: W. W. Norton.
Kelly, Isabel
1955 "El Adiestramiento de Parteras en Mexico, desde el Punto de Vista Antropologica." *América Indígena* 15 (2): 109–17.
Khan, Atiqur Rahman, Farida Akhter Jahan, S. Firoza Begum, and Khalid Jalil
1985 "Maternal Mortality in Rural Bangladesh." *World Health Forum* 6 (4): 325–28.
Kim, Jin-Soon
1987 "Community Health Practitioners in the Republic of Korea." *World Health Forum* 8 (2): 197–99.

Kleinman, Arthur

1978 "International Health Care Planning from an Ethnomedical Perspective: Critique and Recommendations for Change." *Medical Anthropology* 2 (2): 71–96.

1980 *Patients and Healers in the Context of Culture.* Berkeley: University of California Press.

1986 *Social Origins of Distress and Disease.* New Haven: Yale University Press.

Kline, N. S.

1981 "The Endorphins Revisited." *Psychiatric Annals* 11:137–42.

Koss, Joan D.

1975 "Therapeutic Aspects of Puerto Rican Cult Practices." *Psychiatry* 38 (May): 160–70.

1980 "The Therapist-Spiritist Training Project in Puerto Rico: An Experiment to Relate the Traditional Healing System to the Public Health System." *Social Science and Medicine* 14B:255–66.

Kraljevic, I.

1977 *Comisión de Supervisión y Evaluación del Proyecto de Salud Rural—Montero.* Informe Final. La Paz: MPSSP.

1978 "Montero Rural Health Project." Consultant's Report, USAID, Mimeo. Bolivian Mission, La Paz.

Kroeger, A., and E. Luna, eds.

1985 *Atención Primaria de Salud: Guía para Médicos y Enfermeras que Trabajan en Zonas Rurales de Latinoamérica.* Berlin: Deutsche Stiftung für Internationale Entwicklung.

Kunitz, Stephen

1983 *Disease Change and the Role of Medicine: The Navajo Experience.* Berkeley: University of California Press.

Land, Thomas

1986 "Herbal Healing." *The New Leader* 69 (17): 3.

Last, Murray

1986 "The Professionalization of African Medicine: Ambiguities and Definitions." In *The Professionalisation of African Medicine,* edited by M. Last and G. L. Chavunduka, 1–26. Manchester: Manchester University Press.

Leach, Edmund

1976 *Culture and Communication.* Cambridge: Cambridge University Press.

Leslie, Charles

1976 *Asian Medical Systems: A Comparative Study.* Berkeley: University of California Press.

1980 "Medical Pluralism in World Perspective." *Social Science and Medicine* 14B (4): 191–95.

Levi-Strauss, Claude

1967 *Structural Anthropology,* translated by M. Layton. New York: Anchor Books.

Lex, B. W.

1976 "Psychological Aspects of Ritual Trance." *Journal of Altered States of Consciousness* 2:109–22.

1978 "Neurological Bases of Revitalization." *Zygon* 13:276–312.

Lieban, R. W.

1977 "Symbols, Signs and Success: Healers and Power in a Philippine City." In *The Anthropology of Power,* edited by R. D. Fogelson and R. Adams, 57–66. New York: Academic Press.

Lock, Margaret
1987 "Introduction." In *Health, Illness, and Medical Care in Japan*, edited by Edward Norbeck and M. Lock, 1–23. Honolulu: University of Hawaii Press.
1987a "Protests of a Good Wife and Wise Mother: The Medicalization of Distress in Japan." In *Health, Illness, and Medical Care in Japan*, edited by Edward Norbeck and M. Lock, 130–57. Honolulu: University of Hawaii Press.

Low, Setha
1988 "The Medicalization of Healing Cults in Latin America." *American Ethnologist* 15:187.

Luborsky, Lester, Barton Singer, and Lise Luborsky
1975 "Comparative Studies of Psychotherapies." *Archives of General Psychiatry* 32 (8): 995–1008.

Luna, Eduardo
1986 *Vegetalismo: Shamanism among the Mestizo Population of the Peruvian Amazon*. Stockholm: Almqvist & Wiksell.

MacCormack, C.
1986 "The Articulation of Western and Traditional Systems of Health Care." In *The Professionalisation of African Medicine*, edited by M. Last and G. L. Chavunduka, 151–61. Manchester: Manchester University Press.

McElroy, Ann, and Patricia K. Townsend
1985 *Medical Anthropology in Ecological Perspective*. Boulder, Colo.: Westview Press.

McEwen, W.
1975 *Changing Rural Society: A Study of Communities in Bolivia*. New York: Oxford University Press.

Maclean, Una, and Robert Bannerman
1982 "Utilization of Indigenous Healers in National Health Delivery Systems." *Social Science and Medicine* 16:1815–16.

MacLeod, Roy
1988 "Introduction." In *Medicine and Empire: Perspectives on Western Medicine and the Experience of European Expansion*, edited by R. MacLeod and M. Lewis, 1–18. New York: Routledge.

Maddi, Salvatore R.
1976 *Personality Theories: A Comparative Analysis*. 3d ed. Homewood, Ill.: The Dorsey Press.

Mahadevappa, H.
1984 "Community Health Workers—Resources Could Be Better Spent." *World Health Forum* 5 (2): 149–50.

Mandelbaum, D. G.
1974 *Human Fertility in India: Social Components and Policy Perspectives*. Berkeley: University of California Press.

Marcos de Silveira, Claudio, and Percy Halkyer
1988 *Informe sobre el Control de Tétanos Neonatal en Bolivia*. La Paz: UNICEF and PAHO.

Margoulies, Leah
1977 "Exporting Infant Malnutrition." In *Breast versus Bottle: The Scandal of Infant Formula Promotion*, 8–9. Food Monitor Reprint. Garden City, N.Y.: World Hunger Year.

Marshall, Elliot

1980 "Psychotherapy Faces Test of Worth." *Science* 207:35–36.

1980a "Psychotherapy Works, But for Whom?" *Science* 207:506–8.

Maslow, Abraham

1968 *Toward a Psychology of Being.* 2d ed. New York: Van Nostrand Reinhold.

Mburu, F. M.

1977 "The Duality of Traditional and Western Medicine in Africa: Mystics, Myths and Reality." In *Traditional Healing: New Science or New Colonialism?*, edited by Philip Singer, 158–85. Buffalo, N.Y.: Conch Magazine.

Medalie, Jack

1978 "Discussion on Arthur Kleinman's Paper." *Medical Anthropology* 2 (2): 94–96. (See Kleinman 1978)

Mengert, William, and Douglas P. Murphy

1933 "Intra-abdominal Pressures Created by Voluntary Muscular Effort." *Surgery, Gynecology and Obstetrics* 57:745–51.

Montaño Cuéllar, Dolly

1985 "Estudio Descriptivo sobre Tétanos Neonatal durante el Período 1980 a 1984 en el Servicio de Infecciosas." Montero: Hospital de Niños.

Morelli, Rosella, and Eduardo Missoni

1986 "Training Traditional Birth Attendants in Nicaragua." *World Health Forum* 7 (2): 144–49.

Morgan, Lynn M.

1987 "Dependency Theory in the Political Economy of Health: An Anthropological Critique." *Medical Anthropology Quarterly* 1:131–54.

1989 " 'Political Will' and Community Participation in Costa Rican Primary Health Care." *Medical Anthropology Quarterly* 3:232–45.

Morley, D., and H. Lovel

1986 *My Name Is Today: An Illustrated Discussion of Child Health, Society and Poverty in Less Developed Countries.* London: MacMillan.

Mosley, Paul

1987 *Foreign Aid: Its Defense and Reform.* Lexington: University Press of Kentucky.

Mull, J. Dennis

1990 "The Primary Health Care Dialectic: History, Rhetoric, and Reality." In *Anthropology and Primary Health Care*, edited by J. Coreil and J. D. Mull, 28–48. Boulder, Colo.: Westview Press.

Muñoz Reyes, Jorge

1977 *Geografía de Bolivia.* La Paz: Academia Nacional de Ciencias de Bolivia.

Navarro, Vicente

1984 "A Critique of the Ideological and Political Positions of the Willy Brandt Report and the WHO Alma-Ata Declaration." *Social Science and Medicine* 19:467–74.

Nchinda, T. C.

1976 "Traditional and Western Medicine in Africa: Collaboration or Confrontation?" *Tropical Doctor* 6:133–35.

Neher, Andrew

1962 "A Physiological Explanation of Unusual Behavior in Ceremonies Involving Drums." *Human Biology* 34(2): 151–60.

Neumann, Alfred K., Daniel A. Ampofo, David D. Nicholas, Samuel Ofosu-Amaah, and Frederick K. Wurapa

1974 "Traditional Birth Attendants: A Key to Rural Maternal and Child

Health and Family Planning Services." *Environmental Child Health* 20 (February): 21–27.

———, and P. Lauro

1982 "Ethnomedicine and Biomedicine Linking." *Social Science and Medicine* 16:1817–24.

———, Samuel Ofosu-Amaah, Daniel A. Ampofo, David D. Nicholas, and Rexford O. Asante

1976 "Integration of Family Planning and Maternal and Child Health in Rural West Africa." *Journal of Biosocial Science* 8:161–73.

Newell, Kenneth W.

1975 *Health by the People.* Geneva: WHO.

Nicholas, David D., Daniel A. Ampofo, Samuel Ofosu-Amaah, R. O. Asante, and Alfred K. Neumann

1976 "Attitudes and Practices of Traditional Birth Attendants in Rural Ghana: Implications for Training in Africa." *World Health Organization Bulletin* 54:343–48.

Nichols, M. P., and Melvin Zax

1977 *Catharsis in Psychotherapy.* New York: Columbia University Press.

Nichter, Mark

1990 "Vaccinations in South Asia: False Expectations and Commanding Metaphors." In *Anthropology and Primary Health Care,* edited by J. Coreil and J. D. Mull, 196–221. Boulder, Colo.: Westview Press.

Nishimura, Kho

1978 "Shaman Bunka to Seishin Iryo (Shamanistic Culture and Psychiatric Cures)." In *Bunka to Seishinbyori* (Culture and Psychopathology). Tokyo: Kobundo.

1987 "Shamanism and Medical Cures." *Current Anthropology* 28 (4): S59–S64.

Obeyesekere, Gananath

1970 "The Idiom of Demonic Possession." *Social Science and Medicine* 4:97–111.

Oblitas Poblete, Enrique

1968 *La Lengua Secreta de los Incas.* La Paz: Editorial "Los Amigos del Libro."

1969 *Plantas Medicinales en Bolivia.* La Paz: Editorial "Los Amigos del Libro."

1978 *Cultura Callawaya.* La Paz: Imprenta "Alba."

Owen, Margaret, Galba Araujo, J. K. Harfouche, Elton Kessel, Vijay Kumar, Elizabeth Leedam, and Belmont Williams

1983 "Round Table: The Traditional Birth Attendant and the Law." *World Health Forum* 4 (4): 291–312.

Parsons, Talcott

1975 "The Sick Role and the Role of the Physician Reconsidered." *Health and Society* 53 (3): 257–78.

———, and Renee Fox

1975 "Illness, Therapy and the Modern Urban American Family." *Journal of Social Issues* 8:31–44.

Paul, Benjamin, and William J. Demarest

1984 "Citizen Participation Overplanned: The Case of a Health Project in the Guatemalan Community of San Pedro Laguna." *Social Science and Medicine* 19 (3): 185–92.

Paul, Lois

1975 "Recruitment to a Ritual Role: The Midwife in a Maya Community." *Ethos* 3 (3): 449–67.

Paul, Lois, and Benjamin Paul

1975 "The Maya Midwife as a Sacred Specialist: A Guatemalan Case." *American Ethnologist* 2 (4): 707–26.

Pellegrino, Edmund D.

1979 "The Sociocultural Impact of Twentieth-Century Therapeutics." In *The Therapeutic Revolution,* edited by Morris Vogel and Charles E. Rosenberg, 245–66. Philadelphia: University of Pennsylvania Press.

Pfleiderer, Beatrix, and Wolfgang Bichman

1985 *Krankheit und Kultur: Eine Einfuebrung in die Ethno- medizin.* Berlin: Dietrich Reimer Verlag.

Phillips, David R.

1990 *Health and Health Care in the Third World.* New York: John Wiley.

Pillsbury, Barbara

1979 *Reaching the Rural Poor: Indigenous Health Practitioners Are There Already.* Washington, D.C.: USAID.

Pratinidhi, A. K., A. N. Shrotri, Usha Shah, and H. H. Chavan

1985 "Birth Attendants and Perinatal Mortality." *World Health Forum* 6 (2): 115–17.

Pratt, Lois V.

1978 "Reshaping the Consumer's Posture in Health Care." In *The Doctor-Patient Relationship in the Changing Health Scene,* edited by Eugene B. Gallagher, 197–214 DHEW Publication No. (NIH) 78–183. Washington, D.C.: U.S. Department of Health, Education, and Welfare; Public Health Service, National Institute of Health.

Prince, R.

1982 "Shamans and Endorphins: Hypotheses for a Synthesis." *Ethos* 10:409–23.

Project Identification Document (PID)

1988 "Community and Child Health Project (511:0594)." La Paz: Government of Bolivia and USAID.

Raphael, Dana

1976 "Warning: The Milk in This Package May Be Lethal for Your Infant." In *Medical Anthropology,* edited by F. Grollig and H. Haley, 129–36. The Hague: Mouton.

———, ed.

1980 *Breastfeeding and Food Policy in a Hungry World.* New York: Academic Press.

Rasnake, R.

1988 *Domination and Cultural Resistance: Authority and Power among an Andean People.* Durham: Duke University Press.

Rogers, Carl

1980 *A Way of Being.* Boston: Houghton Mifflin.

Rogers, E.

1983 *Diffusion of Innovations.* New York: The Free Press.

Rosenberg, Charles E.

1979 "The Therapeutic Revolution: Medicine, Meaning and Social Change in Nineteenth-Century America." In *The Therapeutic Revolution,* edited by M. J. Vogel and Charles E. Rosenberg, 3–25. Philadelphia: University of Pennsylvania Press.

Rosing, Ina

1990 *Introducción al Mundo Callawaya.* La Paz: "Los Amigos del Libro."

Rowe, John
  1946 "Inca Culture at the Time of the Spanish Conquest." In *Handbook of South American Indians*, vol. 2, edited by J. Steward, 198–330. Washington, D.C.: Smithsonian Institution.
Rubel, Arthur
  1964 "Epidemiology of a Folk Illness: *Susto* in Hispanic America." *Ethnology* 3:268–83.
Rubel, Arthur, Rolando Collado Ardón, Carl W. O'Nell, and Raymond Murray
  1983 "A Folk Illness (Susto) as an Indicator of Real Illness." *The Lancet*, no. 8363 (December 10): 1362.
  1984 *Susto: A Folk Illness.* Berkeley: University of California Press.
Ruiz, P. and J. Langrod
  1976 "The Role of Folk Healers in Community Mental Services." *Community Mental Health Journal* 12 (4): 392–98.
Sai, Fred T., René Dumont, Mohammed Fazlul Haque, Attiya Inayatullah, James T. McHugh, Sat Paul Mittal, Pramilla Senanayake, Haryono Suyono, and J. S. Tomkinson
  1986 "Round Table: Family Planning and Maternal Health Care, a Common Goal." *World Health Forum* 7:315–38.
Saignes, Thierry
  1984 "Quienes Son los Callahuayas? Nota sobre un Enigma Histórico." In *Espacio y Tiempo en el Mundo Callahuaya*, edited by T. Gisbert and P. Seibert, 111–29. La Paz: Universidad Mayor de San Andrés.
Sargent, Carolyn Fishel
  1974 *The Cultural Context of Therapeutic Choice: Obstetrical Care Decisions among the Bariba of Benin.* Boston: Reidel.
Schaedel, R.
  1988 "Andean World View: Hierarchy or Reciprocity, Regulation or Control?" *Current Anthropology* 29 (5): 768–75.
Scheff, T. J.
  1979 *Catharsis in Healing, Ritual, and Drama.* Berkeley: University of California Press.
Scheper-Hughes, Nancy, and Margaret Lock
  1987 "The Mindful Body: A Prolegomenon to Future Work in Medical Anthropology." *Medical Anthropology Quarterly* 1 (1): 6–41.
Schumacher, Ernst
  1987 "Village Midwife Training on Huon Peninsula." *Papua New Guinea Medical Journal* 30:213–17.
Scrimshaw, Susan, and Elizabeth Burleigh
  1978 *The Potential for the Integration of Indigenous and Western Medicines in Latin America and Hispanic Populations in the United States of America.* Scientific Publication no. 359. Washington D.C.: Pan American Health Organization.
Selye, H.
  1956 *The Stress of Life.* New York: McGraw-Hill.
SEMTA (*Servicios Múltiples de Tecnologías Apropiadas*)
  1984 *Plantas y Tratamientos Kallawayas.* La Paz: SEMTA.
Sharon, Doug, and Donald Joralemon
  1987 "Psychosocial Therapy in Peruvian Folk Healing." Progress Report, November, p. 10. Washington D.C.: NIMH.
  1989 "Final Grant Report: Psychosocial Therapy in Peruvian Shamanism," No. MH38685, 1–11. Washington D.C., NIMH.

Shirokogoroff, S. M.
  1935 *Psychomental Complex of the Tungus.* London: Kegan Paul, Trench, Trubner.
Siegler, Miriam, and Humphrey Osmond
  1974 *Models of Madness, Models of Medicine.* New York: MacMillan.
Singer, Philip
  1977 "Introduction." In *Traditional Healing: New Science or New Colonialism?* edited by Philip Singer, 1–25. Buffalo, N.Y.: Conch Magazine.
Slikkerveer, Leendert Jan
  1982 "Rural Health Development in Ethiopia: Problems of Utilization of Traditional Healers." *Social Science and Medicine* 16:1859–72.
Smith, Gavin
  1989 *Livelihood and Resistance: Peasants and the Politics of Land in Peru.* Berkeley: University of California Press.
Smith, Mary Lee, and Gene V. Glass
  1977 "Meta-Analysis of Psychotherapy Outcome Studies." *American Psychologist* 32:752–60.
Snyder, Solomon H.
  1977 "Opiate Receptors and Internal Opiates." *Scientific American* 236 (3): 44–56.
Spalding, Karen
  1973 "Kurakas and Commerce: A Chapter in the Evolution of Andean Society." *Hispanic American Historical Review* 53 (4): 581–99.
Stark, Louisa
  1972 "Machaj-juyai: Secret Language of the Callahuayas." *Papers in Andean Linguistics* 1:199–227.
Starr, Paul
  1982 *The Social Transformation of American Medicine.* New York: Basic Books.
Stein, Howard F.
  1990 *American Medicine as Culture.* Boulder, Colo.: Westview Press.
Steltzer, Ulli
  1983 *Health in the Guatemalan Highlands.* Seattle: University of Washington Press.
Strupp, Hans H.
  1980 "Success and Failure in Time-Limited Psychotherapy." *Archives of General Psychiatry* 37:708–16, 831–41, 947–54.
Stycos, J. M.
  1968 *Human Fertility in Latin America: Sociological Perspectives.* Ithaca: Cornell University Press.
Sullivan, Lawrence E.
  1987 "Healing." In *Encyclopedia of Religion,* edited by M. Eliade, vol. 6, 226–34. New York: Macmillan Publishing Company.
Susser, Mervy
  1974 "Ethical Components in the Definition of Health." *International Journal of Health Services* 4:539–48.
Tan, Michael L.
  1988 "Primary Health Care and Indigenous Medicine." *Cultural Survival Quarterly* 12 (1): 8–10.
Thomas, Lewis
  1977 "On the Science and Technology of Medicine." *Daedalus* 106:35–46.
Torrey, E. G.
  1973 *Witchdoctors and Psychiatrists.* New York: Bantam Books.

Torrico Espinoza, Gloria
  1987 "Incidencia de Pacientes con Tétanos Neonatal en el Año 1985."
    Unpub. ms. Montero: Hospital de Niños.
Ugalde, Antonio
  1985 "Ideological Dimensions of Community Participation in Latin
    American Health Programs." *Social Science and Medicine* 21 (1): 41–53.
UNITAS
  1988 *El Alto desde El Alto.* Documentos de Análisis 5. La Paz.
Valdizán, H., and Angel Maldonado
  1922 *La Medicina Popular Peruana.* 3 vols. Lima: Imprenta Torres Aguirre.
van Binsbergen, Wim
  1988 "The Land as Body: An Essay on the Interpretation of Ritual among
    the Manjaks of Guinea-Bissau." *Medical Anthropology Quarterly* 2 (4):
    386–401.
van den Berg, Hans
  1990 *La Tierra No Da Asi Nomas: Los Ritos Agrícolas en la Religión de los Aymara-
    Cristianos.* La Paz: Hisbol-UCB/ISET.
van den Berghe, Pierre, and George Primov
  1977 *Inequality in the Peruvian Andes: Class and Ethnicity in the Cuzco Area.*
    Columbia: University of Missouri Press.
Van Gennep, Arnold
  1960 *Rites of Passage.* Chicago: University of Chicago Press.
Van Schaik, Eileen
  1989 "Paradigms Underlying the Study of Nerves as a Popular Illness Term
    in Eastern Kentucky." *Medical Anthropology* 2:15–28.
Vansintejan, Gilberte, and Robin C. Davis
  1986 "A Training Initiative for Community Health Workers in Rural Haiti."
    World Health Forum 7 (2): 150–53.
Velimirovic, Boris
  1990 "Is Integration of Traditional and Western Medicine Really Possible?"
    In *Anthropology and Primary Health Care,* edited by J. Coreil and J. D.
    Mull, 51–78. Boulder, Colo.: Westview Press.
Wachtel, N.
  1973 "La Reciprocidad y el Estado Inca: De Karl Polanyi a John V. Murra." In
    Sociedad e Ideología, edited by N. Wachtel, 59–78. Lima: Instituto de
    Estudios Peruanos.
Wagley, Charles
  1977 *Welcome of Tears: The Tapirape Indians of Central Brazil.* New York: Oxford
    University Press.
Warren, Dennis W., G. S. Bova, M. A. Tregoning, and Mark Kliewer
  1982 "Ghanian National Policy towards Indigenous Healers: The Case of
    the Primary Health Training for Indiginous Healers (PRHETIH) Pro-
    gram." *Social Science and Medicine* 16 (21): 1873–82.
_____, and Edward C. Green
  1988 "Linking Biomedical and Indigenous African Health Delivery Sys-
    tems: An Assessment of Collaborative Efforts during the 1980s." In
    Symposium of Ethnomedical Systems in Sub-Saharan Africa, 1–10. African
    Studies Center, Leiden, the Netherlands, June.
Wassén, Henry
  1972 *A Medicine-man's Implements and Plants in a Tiahuanacoid Tomb in High-
    land Bolivia.* Goteborg: Goteborgs Etnografiska Museum.

Welsch, R. L.
1988 "Primary Health Care: A Papua New Guinea Example." *Cultural Survival Quarterly* 12 (1): 1–4.

Werner, David
1977 *Where There Is No Doctor: A Village Health Care Handbook.* Palo Alto, Calif.: Hesperian Foundation.
1981 *Donde No Hay Doctor.* Palo Alto, Calif.: Hesperian Foundation.
————, and Bill Bower
1982 *Helping Health Workers Learn.* Palo Alto, Calif.: Hesperian Foundation.

Werner, Richard
1980 "Deception and Self-Deception in Shamanism and Psychiatry." *International Journal of Social Psychiatry* 26:41–52.

Willis, W. D., H. Akil, A. I. Babaum, J. M. Besson, E. Carstens, K. L. Casey, B. L. Finer, A. Herz, V. Höllt, A. Iggo, H. Takagi, and W. Zieglgänsberger
1979 "Central Mechanisms of Pain Control." In *Pain and Society,* edited by H. W. Kosterlitz and L. Y. Terenius, 239–62. Weinheim: Verlag Chemie.

Wittkower, E. D.
1970 "Trance and Possession States." *International Journal of Social Psychiatry* 16 (2): 153–60.

Wolf, Eric
1985 "Types of Latin American Peasantry: A Preliminary Discussion." *American Anthropologist* 52:452–55.

Wood, Corinne Shear
1990 "Maori Community Health Workers: A Mixed Reception in New Zealand." In *Anthropology and Primary Health Care,* edited by J. Coreil and J. D. Mull, 123–36. Boulder, Colo.: Westview Press.

World Health Organization (WHO)
1965 *International Classification of Diseases.* 8th ed. Geneva: WHO.
1977 *Committee A: Provisional Record of the 18th Meeting (World Health Organization).* Thirtieth World Health Assembly. A30/A/SR/18. Geneva: WHO.
1978 *The Promotion and Development of Traditional (or Indigenous) Medicine Programme.* Technical Report Series no. 622. Geneva: WHO.
1987 *Neonatal Tetanus Elimination: AFRO Is Taking the Lead Position.* WHO/ EPI/GAG. Geneva: WHO.
———— and Expanded Program on Immunization (EPI). Global Advisory Group.
1991 *Progress on the Global Plan for NNT Elimination.* EPI/GAG/W.P. 10 (October). Antalya, Turkey.
————, and United Nations International Children's Emergency Fund (UNICEF)
1978 *Primary Health Care: A Joint Report by the Director-General of the World Health Organization and the Executive Director of the United Nations Children's Fund.* Geneva-New York: WHO.

Yoder, P. Stanley
1982 "Biomedical and Ethnomedical Practice in Rural Zaire: Contrasts and Complements." *Social Science and Medicine* 16:1851–57.

Young, Alan.
1977 "Order, Analogy and Efficacy in Ethiopian Medical Divination." *Culture, Medicine, and Psychiatry* 1:183–99.
1982 "The Anthropologies of Illness and Sickness." In *Annual Review of*

Anthropology, edited by B. Siegel, 257–85. Palo Alto, Calif.: Annual Reviews.

Young, James C.
1981 *Medical Choice in a Mexican Village.* New Brunswick: Rutgers University Press.

Zola, I. K.
1978 "Medicine as an Institution of Social Control." In *The Cultural Crisis of Modern Medicine,* edited by J. Ehrenreich, 80–100. New York: Monthly Review Press.

Zuidema, R. T.
1964 *The Ceque System of Cuzco: The Social Organization of the Capital of the Inca.* Leiden: Brill.

Index

Abortion, 164
Agpasa, Tony, 216
Agriculture, 48–49, 131–32
Ajayu, 181, 203
Alma-Ata report, 4, 5, 6, 18
Altiplano, 201–6
Alvarez, Florentine, 38–39, 47, 58–63, 71, 184
Alvarez, Walter, 57, 61, 62
Amaringo, Pablo, 84
Anemia, 164
Antiseptic practices, 141, 179–80
Anthropology, 227–28. *See also* Medical anthropology
Apprenticeship, 58. *See also* Education; Training
Articulation model, 39–43
Associations, ethnomedical, 99–101, 229–30
Autonomy, ethnomedical practitioners, 37–38, 221–22
Ayahuasca, 77
Aymara, 201–6, 212
Ayllu, 48–49, 118, 127, 128
Ayni (exchange), 130–31
Ayurvedic medicine, 20

Bangladesh, 22, 194–96, 212
Baptism, 210
Barter, 131
Bastien, Joseph, 19, 24, 31, 162–63
Behrhorst, Carroll, 105–10
Bhuts, 195
Biomedical and ethnomedical practitioners. *See also* Community health workers; Diviners; Doctors; Herbalists; Midwives; Nurses; Shamans and shamanism
clinics, 188–91
collaboration between, 181–83, 218–23, 227–35
culturally defined illnesses, 183–87
experiences of illnesses, 176–81
health records, 223–25

obstacles to integration of, 33–36
referrals, 225–27
treatment of *susto*, 181–83
workshops with, 174–76, 187–88
Biomedicine. *See also* Ethnomedicine
adaptive strategies of Bolivian herbalists to, 47–71
cultural adaptation and community health worker programs, 136
deficiencies of in primary health care, 3–18
government policy and articulation model of integration, 41–43
medical trends of present and future, 215
midwives and integration, 138–39, 161
shamans and, 75–76, 77, 93–94, 95–96
theories of integration, 36–41
Birth control. *See* Family planning
Birth-control pills, 165
Bolivia. *See also* Aymara; Kallawaya; Quechua; Tupi-Guarani
adaptive strategies of herbalists to biomedicine, 47–71
alternative medical traditions, 20–21
autonomy model of medical integration, 38
clinics with ethnomedical and biomedical practitioners, 188–91
community health-worker programs, 108, 110, 112–36
economics and access to biomedicine, 13, 15–16
ethnomedical and biomedical practitioners and experience of illnesses, 176–81
example of collaboration between biomedical and ethnomedical practitioners, 233–35
family planning, 162–63

259